SUCCESSFUL SURGICAL RESEARCH –
How to Plan, Perform and Publish

Editors
Kemal I. Deen, MD, MS, FRCS
Professor and Chair of Surgery, University of Kelaniya Medical
School, Sri Lanka

&

Ravin R. Kumar, MD, FRCS, FACS, FASCRS
Assistant Professor of Surgery at David Geffen School of Medicine
at University College of Los Angeles
Chief, Division of Colon and Rectal Surgery
Harbor-UCLA Medical Center
Torrance, California, USA

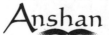

Anshan Limited, (UK)

Anshan Limited
6 Newlands Road
Tunbridge Wells
Kent TN4 9AT, UK
Tel/Fax : + 44 (0) 1892 557767
e-mail : infor@anshan.co.uk
Website : www.anshan.co.uk

British Library Cataloguing in Publication Data
A catalogue record for this book is available from the British Library.

Not for sale in India, Pakistan, Nepal, Sri Lanka and Bangladesh

ISBN: 1 904 798 71 3
ISBN 978 190 479 871 2

This edition is co-pulished by B.I. Publications Pvt. Ltd. and Anshan Limited, and printed at Saurabh Printers Pvt. Ltd., Noida, India.

List of Contributors

M. H. J. Ariyaratne, MS, FRCS, FRCSE
Senior Lecturer in Surgery, University of Kelaniya Medical School,
Sri Lanka

Christine E. Dauphine, MD
Chief Resident in General Surgery
Harbor-UCLA Medical Center
Torrance, California, USA

Kemal I. Deen, MD, MS, FRCS
Professor and Chair of Surgery, University of Kelaniya Medical
School, Sri Lanka

H. J. de Silva, MD, D Phil (Oxon), FRCP
Professor of Medicine and Dean of the Medical School,
Faculty of Medicine, University of Kelaniya, Sri Lanka
Editor, *Ceylon Medical Journal*

Christian De Virgilio, MD, FACS
Professor of Surgery at David Geffen School of Medicine at
University College of Los Angeles
Vice Chair, Surgery Education
Director, General Surgery Residency Program
Harbor-UCLA Medical Center
Torrance, California, USA

F. R. Fernando, MS, FRCS
Senior Lecturer and Head, Department of Surgery, University of
Kelaniya Medical School,
Sri Lanka

C. Goonaratne, FRCP, PhD
Emeritus Professor of Physiology, Faculty of Medicine, University
of Colombo, Sri Lanka
Editor, *Ceylon Medical Journal*

Jason S. Haukoos, MD, MS
Assistant Professor
Division of Emergency Medicine
Department of Surgery
Division of Epidemiology and Community Health
Department of Preventive Medicine and Biometrics
University of Colorado Health Sciences Center
Denver, Colorado, USA

Michael R. B. Keighley, MS, FRCS
Barling Professor of Surgery (Emeritus), University of
Birmingham Medical School
United Kingdom
Visiting Professor of Surgery, the Christian Medical College,
Vellore, India

Viken R. Konyalian, MD
Chief Resident in General Surgery
Harbor-UCLA Medical Center
Torrance, California, USA

Ravin R. Kumar, MD, FRCS, FACS, FASCRS
Assistant Professor of Surgery at David Geffen School of Medicine
at University College of Los Angeles
Chief, Division of Colon and Rectal Surgery
Harbor-UCLA Medical Center
Torrance, California, USA

Stewart A. Laidlaw, PhD
Professor of Medicine, David Geffen School of Medicine, UCLA
Director, Compliance and Regulatory Affairs,
Director, Educational Outreach
Los Angeles Biomedical Research Institute at Harbor-UCLA
Medical Center
Torrance, California, USA

Jason T. Lee, MD
Fellow in Vascular Surgery
Stanford University
Palo Alto, California, USA

R. Navaratnam, MSc, MS, FRCS
Consultant Colorectal Surgeon, The North Middlesex Hospital,
London, United Kingdom

A. Pathmeswaran, MD
Senior Lecturer in Community Medicine, University of Kelaniya
Medical School, Sri Lanka.

M. T. P. R. Perera, MS
Senior Resident in Surgery
The University Surgical Unit at North Colombo General Hospital,
Ragama, Sri Lanka

A. H. Sheriffdeen, FRCS, FRCSE
Professor of Surgery, Emeritus
Department of Surgery, Faculty of Medicine
University of Colombo, Sri Lanka

S. V. Shrikhande, MS
Assistant Professor of Gastrointestinal Surgery, The Tata Memorial
Hospital
Mumbai, India

P. J. Shukla, MS, FRCS
Associate Professor and Chief of Gastrointestinal Surgery, The
Tata Memorial Hospital
Mumbai, India

M. A. Silva, MS, FRCSE
Lecturer in Surgery, University of Kelaniya Medical School, Sri
Lanka
and
Liver Transplant Fellow, The Queen Elizabeth Hospital,
Birmingham, United Kingdom

Bruce E. Stabile, MD, FACS
Professor of Surgery at David Geffen School of Medicine at
University College of Los Angeles
Chairman, Department of Surgery
Harbor-UCLA Medical Center
Torrance, California, USA

A. R. Wickremasinghe, PhD
Professor of Community Medicine, University of Kelaniya Medical
School, Sri Lanka

S. R. E. Wijesuriya, MS
Lecturer in Surgery, University of Kelaniya Medical School, Sri
Lanka

Foreword 1

Surgical research by academic surgeons! Are these not an endangered species of cranks, perceived by the diehard cutters as irrelevant and their competence with a knife under suspicion? What relevance do they have in saving lives? Plenty — you will discover. Surgeons with an interest in research are only an endangered species in those parts of the world that have lost their vision, where clinical practice has been strangled by administrators obsessed by performance indicators and driven by tick boxes. Research is the breath of all clinical endeavour; without it, we wither on the vine, because research is the process of questioning what we do today and inspires change for tomorrow. Society that has temporarily jettisoned research in surgery will stagnate until it recognizes that the dry, arid soil of the treadmill of service encourages no growth. Surgical society needs individuals who will galvanize the rains that germinate a seed of endeavour, discovery and improved clinical practice.

A book at the beginning of the 21st century to guide the formative researcher in surgery is timely. Research in surgery is becoming a curricular requirement in many countries which have accepted the need to provide trainees with an opportunity to discover the dimension of research within the bound of clinical work.

Surgical research can involve very different skills. Only a few leave the clinical arena altogether to enter the laboratory world and engage in P.C.R., Eliza assays or G.L.C. More commonly, the laboratory is the link to correlate clinical data with the science of laboratory measurement. Increasingly, surgeons lead the field of the randomized trial to compare one treatment against no treatment or alternative therapy.

This book takes the embryo surgical researcher, temporarily away from the ward and the operating room, through the process of research planning, particularly the protocol (a research business plan) for the ethical committee submission to the project and its publication. The reader is provided with comprehensive advice about setting up a research project. There are good tips about time management and the contract of a research protocol that is likely to succeed if succinctly described. The need to read, collaborate, communicate and deliver is emphasized by many of the contributors. The special relationship between the research fellow and the supervisor is described as well as the discipline of planning, filing, record keeping and networking.

There is an excellent chapter on the statistical method which is a "must" for all those planning their project and analyzing the results. The reader will have no difficulty in understanding the importance of data distribution, variability, power, type I and type II errors, sensitivity, specificity, positive and negative predictive values, linear regression and survival analysis.

When the data have been gathered, recruitment is over and the study closed, the research has only just begun! This book informs the reader that research without publication is a failure. The "object of science is publication," "work, finish, publish" are the quotes. Successful publication requires more statistics, and the commitment to produce the draft paper before it is torn to shreds by local peer review prior to submission to the journals. The importance of clear writing, tables, updating bibliography and, above all, an eye catching abstract is emphasized by the authors.

This book will be an invaluable compendium to all surgeons who explore the, at times frustrating but eventually rewarding, world of research in surgery. The ethical issues, administrative hurdles, transparency and commitment to the task of exploring the hypothesis and publishing the findings are comprehensively described. Above all, the text emphasizes the importance of integrity in research publication, particularly the avoidance of plagiarism, fraud and unnecessary publication.

The text with its international lineup of experts will prove to be an invaluable acquisition for the trainee planning to undertake research or for the established surgeon inspired to make the clinical laboratory of every day practice a research opportunity.

Michael R. B. Keighley, MS, FRCS
Barling Professor of Surgery (Emeritus)
University of Birmingham Medical School
United Kingdom

Foreword 2

In the United States and some other countries, a nascent concern regarding the future viability of academic surgery has prompted much professional introspection and a call-to-arms for the reinvention of surgical training. The fiscal stability of medical schools and teaching hospitals has become increasingly imperiled by inadequate government support, declining insurance payments, an increasing proportion of uninsured patients, and the ever rising costs of modern medical care. As a result, academic Departments of Surgery and their faculties have been required to increase clinical productivity in order to subsidize both medical education and institutional overhead costs. Academic surgeons now must devote an overwhelming majority of their time and effort to compensatable clinical care in order to sustain their departments, hospitals and schools, as well as their personal incomes. Not surprisingly, medical education and surgical research have become the principal victims of this deleterious paradigm shift.

Funding for surgical research has also declined and the level of competition for scarce resources has escalated substantially. For academic surgery to continue to survive, young surgeons must work more smartly and more efficiently than ever before to achieve success as basic science or clinical investigators. This will require new levels of knowledge and sophistication in the methodology of scientific inquiry, as well as a deep commitment to the ideals of academic surgery.

This book of surgical research is intended to be a primer for young students of surgery who aspire to careers in academic surgery and surgical research. The book is truly international in its editorship and authorship and is intended to provide a concise yet comprehensive distillation of all the essential components necessary for the conduct of surgical research, from planning to presentation and publication. The chapters are arranged in a sequence to usher the reader through the entire process and include both broad overview and practical detail in abundance. The authors include largely American and Sri Lankan surgeons who are actively engaged in the conduct, supervision, editorial review and publication of surgical research. Their collective experience and expertise are invaluable to the novice investigator and it is our hope that the concepts and information provided will serve as a useful guide and facilitator for the launching of many a successful and fulfilling career in academic surgery.

Bruce E. Stabile, MD, FACS

Professor and Chair
Department of Surgery
Harbor-UCLA Medical Center
Torrance, California, USA

Preface

During our initial days as trainees in surgery, we felt the lack of a single comprehensive guide that would steer us through the uncharted area of a research job and, yet, help us emerge unscathed. This work aims to fill such a void.

The book is intended to help the novice in research get off the blocks and maintain a straight course with an end in sight. With this aim in view, we have included broad overviews of how to plan and conduct research, methods of contemporary research and how to deal with the completed project.

We have been fortunate to be able to draw contributions from a number of research scientists, all of whom have medical background, and, more importantly, are currently active in training programs which involve research. Whilst a multi-author text has its own problems of style, each chapter has been written by truly international experts with a single aim in mind — to keep the flames of surgical research alive. We are grateful to each of our contributors.

This book is intended for both undergraduate and postgraduate researchers in medicine and surgery. We also believe it would be an excellent companion to senior physicians seeking to re-familiarize themselves with current research techniques.

We wish to record our appreciation of all our teachers at the Peradeniya Medical School for helping us develop the inquisitive mind, our parents and families, who, on numerous occasions, have had to put up with idiosyncrasies that are commonplace amongst research workers. Finally, we thank our publishers for their patience and unstinted support.

Kemal I. Deen   **Ravin R. Kumar**

Contents

From Basic Idea to Publication

A. H. Sheriffdeen

Introduction

Research is an exercise or experiment which aims to find a truthful answer to a question. Results of research are now categorized into three levels, based on the evidence gathered. Class or Level I means that there is sufficient evidence that a procedure is effective and useful. Class or Level II indicates conflicting evidence or difference of opinion as to usefulness of the procedure. Class or Level III means that there is no evidence, and general agreement that the procedure is not useful or effective or may even be harmful. Doctors, being scientists by training and professionals in conduct, usually undertake research to satisfy an enquiring mind or to satisfy a desire to invent or innovate. Some, however, may undertake research for personal reasons like career advancement or to embellish curriculum vitae!

Types of Research

Basic research is mostly analytical and is usually applicable to non-clinical subjects, e.g. composition of synovial fluid in osteoarthritis. **Applied research,** in contrast, is usually relevant to a clinical setting. Applied research could be either observational or experimental in nature.

[i] *Observational* research comprises *descriptive* studies like audits and surveys in populations, e.g. incidence of abdominal aortic aneurysms in a sample of over 65-year old population in a given area, or *analytical* studies like the impact of a single intervention in a

community on one occasion (*cross-sectional*) or over a period of time (*longitudinal*).

[ii] *Experimental* studies involve clinical trials in the community or in a hospital or a single unit in a hospital including randomized clinical trials.

The Beginning

The source of inspiration for an idea comes only with a thorough knowledge of the subject. Ideas may arise from discussion with superiors or whilst reading the literature or its references. Perusing books of abstracts often gives the reader ideas to pursue. Such ideas may be original (rare). One can also often re-do research to confirm that findings are applicable in a local setting or look at some aspect not investigated earlier.

Reading and thinking about this idea should bring to one's mind clear objectives or goals. "Why am I going to undertake this study? What am I planning to achieve?" One should not say to oneself "let's do this and see what happens", which is invariably a waste of time. Further review of the literature, discussions with superiors and others interested in the subject will set the stage for the next step – **the development of a protocol**.

- Example of identification of an objective – A study comparing laparoscopic cholecystectomy and minilap cholecystectomy. *General objective* – evaluation as safe and effective operation. *Specific objectives* - time for discharge, time to return to work, cost savings, etc.

Developing the Protocol

Once general and specific objectives are identified, one should look at the target population and the variables that could influence outcome, e.g. age, sex, BMI, co-morbid illnesses, stage of the disease, etc. In addition to these demographic and clinical characteristics, geographical location of residence may influence follow-up. These considerations are vital when one is in pursuit of a truthful answer. It is important, therefore, that at every stage from then onwards a close watch is kept for possible sources of error and appropriate measures taken to safeguard against error. Regular dialogue with a senior experienced investigator helps.

Methodology and Design

Choosing the study subjects

Formulate inclusion and exclusion criteria so that conclusions could be generalized, e.g. those unable to return for follow-up should be excluded, but those who cannot give up smoking for example in a study of intermittent claudication could be included, if equal numbers could be recruited to each arm – if not, they are better excluded.

The help of a statistician to determine the sample size helps at this stage. One of the most important questions one should be prepared to answer is the percentage outcome in the published data and the expected outcome from the experiment. Inadequate sample size is one of the commonest causes of poor research projects.

Study design

This includes the population under study, recruitment, assembling of patient groups or cohorts, allocation for the experiment or treatment, randomization, blinding, measurements/observations or investigations and collection of data.

Unless attention is paid to detail, and every aspect of the study is gone through with each subject in the identical manner, numerous pitfalls and errors could creep into the study. Patient compliance is a key factor. The primary objective is to eliminate bias and chance.

Technical factors

a) Randomization could be done by several methods; the most popular method involves use of random allocation charts with numbers in sealed envelopes.

b) Blinding could be difficult and, if possible, should be applied to patient and assessor. For example, in a study comparing laparoscopic cholecystectomy with minilap cholecystectomy, researchers use simulated blood stained dressings at imaginary port sites in the minilap group to blind the assessing nurses.

c) The measurement should be accurate, consistent and reproducible, e.g. the thickness of cuff and site of application should be specified when measuring the ankle/brachial pressure index in trials on occlusive arterial disease of limbs.

d) Data collection forms should be clear and precise. These must have been pre-tested, especially if there are questions to be answered by patients. Any translations should be checked for accuracy. The entries should be periodically validated by a senior person throughout the project to check accuracy. Pre-testing is a useful exercise; select and train data collectors, pre-test the form by testing their ability to enter data whilst ensuring that all patients understand the questions.

The Project Proposal

A project proposal is now written. This should have a title, names of investigators and supervisors, the introduction and the objectives, methodology and design, and the method of analysis. Necessary forms and safeguards against adverse effects must be included. One should also incorporate a proposed budget, if one is looking for sources of funding. Most agencies do not provide funds for equipment or salaries for the supervisor and principal researcher. It is often useful to have your proposal read by some others to check for clarity.

Ethical Clearance

The proposal should now be sent for ethical clearance. One should state clearly the benefits to every patient included in either arm of the study. This could be difficult when a placebo is used in one arm.

The Research Project

Select the sample from the population using appropriate criteria, having decided on how many the research team could take on each day or in each week. Enter baseline variables into questionnaire, randomize, blind as many sites as possible, apply the interventions or treatment procedure as specified, arrange for regular follow-up (devise methods of reminding or retrieving those who fail to come), measure the outcomes until the end point (as stated in the protocol) is reached.

Processing Data

Once the project has been completed and data have been collected and categorized, it is time to analyze the findings. Appropriate statistical tests (with the concurrence of a statistician) are carried out and validated for statistical significance. The results should be studied keeping the objectives in mind. Any secondary data available should also be analyzed. All adverse effects should be clearly recorded and reported.

Results and Discussion

The results so obtained could be tabulated and studied to determine whether the objectives have been achieved. The data given in the introduction would now form the basis of the discussion stating clearly the significant findings and their comparisons with the data available in the literature. The limitations of the study should be stated, e.g. poor sample size, cohorts not represented in the population under study, non-availability of certain investigations or measurements, etc. Finally, the conclusions should be listed to announce the outcome of the study. This is followed by acknowledgements and references.

References

1. Sivagnanasundaram C. *Learning Research*. 1st ed. Colombo: Print Graphics; 1999.
2. Hulley S B, Cummings S R. *Designing Clinical Research*. 1st ed. Baltimore: Williams and Wilkins; 1988.
3. Pollock A, Evans M. *Surgical Audit*. 1st ed. London: Butterworth & Co; 1989.
4. Pocock S J. *Clinical Trials*. 1st ed. Chicester: John Wiley & Sons; 1984.
5. Guidelines for Clinicians Entering Research. Oxford: Published on behalf of the Academic Medicine Group by the Royal College, Oxprint; 1997.

2

Charting the Course of Your Research

M. A. Silva

Securing a career in academic surgery requires forethought and a burning desire to succeed. Success in one's research job, however, also mandates honesty, strict discipline, creating opportunities, and getting and maintaining support from one's mentors and colleagues. Choosing the most suitable research job that would best advance one's career also plays a role in success in research. This could be a pure research-based job or a job with provision for continued clinical exposure. For a surgical trainee, the ideal would be to have some clinical exposure, since in addition to being better for funding subsistence, it helps overcome the rather irrational fear of the risk of becoming 'deskilled' following a 2-3 year break from surgery.

Basic science research has always been the cornerstone of a solid academic career, even for surgeons. There exists a perception that fellow academicians view surgeons as operating room technicians incapable of laboratory research.[1] Therefore, the collaboration between surgeons and basic scientists is more essential than ever, not only because society still optimally rewards science that has potential clinical applicability,[2] but also because it is the basis for undertaking a research job in the first place. Having a research degree builds one's curriculum vitae and improves the chances of future employability, and this is a driving force behind its need presently.[3] It also results in the advancement of academic surgery and produces clinicians with a long standing commitment to research. This should be borne in mind when starting off on an academic job.

Starting an Academic Job – The Transition

The transition from a busy surgical routine to a research job requires getting used to. From the strict routines (with little or no free time) and the stress of clinical surgery, one faces a sudden transition to a job that does not seem to have any boundaries. Steering one's course in an academic job is very much an individual endeavour. Other than an academic supervisor, there is no one to answer to and it is very much up to the individual how he spends the hours of the day. Suddenly, there seems to be adequate time to catch up with mundane chores that have been shelved during the course of the previous clinical job. Reporting to work as early or as late as one desires does not seem to be an issue. Beware! Weeks soon begin to stretch into months with very little research work being done.

The absence of a clinical commitment and operative exposure will be another change to cope with. The authority and fulfillment a clinical job brings abruptly disappear. A feeling of despair, self-doubt and even disinterest in the new working environment may creep in. Overcoming this is best done by active planning, setting up and commencing one's research. Having a clinical commitment while doing an academic job and attending clinical meetings with relevance to one's interest and research may also help.

Time Management

Time management plays a vital role in the success of a research job.[4] Recognizing this at the onset of the research job is even more important. Spending time with one's supervisor and planning the course of study with realistic time schedules is a critical step. After a broad outline of a research schedule is planned, it is important to further subdivide time intervals. Setting up the study takes up a lot of effort and time. This is usually needed for local and regional ethics committee approvals, registering with a university for a higher degree, setting up accounts for funds, calling for quotations and ordering equipment and consumables.

With the paper work for setting up a project done, a considerable amount of time is spent waiting for committees to meet and approve or suggest amendments to the submitted applications. This could take months if careful planning is not done ahead of time. The time spent in waiting for approvals is a vital period to get familiarized with one's project and laboratory or the clinical techniques needed in the study. Writing a review article is the best possible way to familiarize oneself with a topic. Developing filing systems, creating databases and setting up reference managers using programs like *Endnote* and *Reference Manager* should be done at the onset of a project. Additionally, most research centres have databases with invaluable records. Getting involved early in relevant clinical trials, either retrospective or prospective, is also important for developing an understanding of research methodology and experimental design.

Investing in a personal digital organizer or a diary is money well spent. This helps to plan out a daily schedule ahead of time and to set deadlines. Keeping to deadlines and keeping one's supervisor aware of them is important. Strict self-discipline is an important facet of research and a vital requirement. Similarly, schedules should be drawn up for data collection, laboratory work, data analysis and writing up one's thesis.

Identifying time wasting exercises is also as important as good time management. This too is best achieved early during the setting-up phase of a research project. Integrating a clinical commitment into the program too needs planning. It is always an advantage to have a fixed clinical commitment so that the remainder of your schedule could be planned out rather than working on an ad hoc basis, which could be disruptive and lead to time wastage.

Developing Confidence

Familiarization with laboratory techniques is a challenging task for the clinical trainee with no previous experience. Laboratory staff usually comprises career scientists, technicians and postgraduate students. Finding your way around the laboratory and learning experimental techniques are time consuming and require the help and support of the laboratory staff. Early attempts at experiments are fraught with failure and this is a difficult period to get through. It is important to develop confidence in the techniques and procedures required for research prior to commencing data collection. The initial setting-up phase is also best used to overcome this obstacle.

Abstracts and Closing Dates

With the research project up and running, reviewing of early data is best done in consultation with one's supervisor and experienced colleagues. An introduction to the scientific community is best achieved by presenting on-going work at relevant scientific meetings. Preparing abstracts requires training and this is best achieved by submitting as many as possible. Being aware of closing dates for abstract submissions is critical. Checking the websites of relevant professional societies and registering with those which regularly provide updates on deadlines for abstract submissions is helpful. Generally, a single abstract could be submitted to a local or regional meeting, a national and an international meeting. This gives one maximum mileage and provides much needed experience of presentations at scientific meetings. Be it a local, regional, national or an international meeting, preparation should always be meticulous with regard to content, timing of presentations and managing questions during discussion. It is advantageous to present one's data and papers at weekly laboratory meetings that are usually attended by colleagues and supervisors. This helps in building confidence, keeping presentation within stipulated time period and answering questions that may be posed at a future scientific meeting.

Writing Papers on the Job

Converting presentations into publications is another skill that requires development. This is an indicator which highlights an individual's progress in an academic environment and which is also vital for building good curriculum vitae. For acquiring the skills required to write a scientific paper, one needs practice. Conducting a scientific literature search, learning the basics of statistics and its applications, establishing a clear and plausible message in a scientific paper, writing it, having it reviewed by colleagues and supervisors and making repeated corrections to the text are time consuming activities. Finding the time to fit these into a schedule which already has a laboratory and, if applicable, a clinical commitment also requires planning. Dedicating a fixed number of hours for this purpose each day or week is the only feasible method of achieving the goal.

Submitting a scientific paper to the most appropriate journal for publication is also of importance. A journal related to the subspeciality of one's research is usually appropriate. Selection among journals of the same subspeciality is best done on the basis of their impact factors. Having an article accepted for publication in a journal with the highest possible impact factor is the obvious choice. Articles which are submitted for publication are frequently rejected by editors of journals after peer review. Rejected articles are usually returned with comments made by the reviewers. Most of the criticism an article receives in this setting is constructive and justified. Making amendments to an article according to the suggestions made by reviewers generally contributes towards its eventually getting published, albeit in another journal, which may have a lower impact factor.

A basic understanding of research methodology and experimental design equips the surgical trainee with the ability to understand and critically review medical and surgical literature. Universities commonly hold workshops on evidence-based medicine, which offer training in the skills of reading a scientific article with a view to understanding and developing the ability to identify the merits and demerits of a paper. These are invaluable and are not to be missed. Joining a journal club also helps in this regard while also keeping one abreast of scientific developments in one's field.

Meeting with Supervisor – Continued Need for Mentorship

Chair support and collaboration with peers and mentors have been identified as factors contributing to success in a research job.[5] Regular meetings with your supervisor and research group also ensure that deadlines are met. Discussions on progress and projected targets are usual at such meeting. More often than not in scientific research, experiments may go wrong. Regular research group meeting always help one share experience and identify mistakes. Communication with colleagues, especially those with greater experience in the field of research and experimental techniques is useful. It is also the duty of the researcher to keep one's supervisor informed of scheduled experiments, approaching meetings, presentations and delicate matters such as authorship to papers. Relationship with one's supervisor must be maintained as cordial as possible at all times.

Developing Philosophy of Academic Growth

One objective of having competency to appropriately examine scientific knowledge is to enable the surgical trainee to objectively evaluate and apply scientific advances and new treatments in the management of patients. Participation in research also provides the trainee an opportunity to contribute new medical and surgical knowledge and techniques to scientific literature. Research activities also enhance the ability to link research results with clinical activities. Academic surgeons have always been involved in teaching surgical trainees in some capacity. Thus, the philosophy of academic growth while on the job augers well for the future of surgical training in general.

Intellectual and Emotional Honesty

Maintaining the integrity of affiliated institutes is a necessary prerequisite in an academic career. This is of importance, especially when generating results in a research project. All efforts must be made to ensure accuracy of data entry and statistical analysis. It is always good to have one's calculations checked by an independent source having a mathematical and statistical background. Care should also be taken not to infringe on copyright laws. Regulations regarding publications must be studied and followed always. Maintaining accurate records, which are reproducible and devising filing systems which are readily accessible help avoid inaccuracies.

Myths, Mental and Physical Health

Taking time off clinical surgery to pursue training in research is believed, rather irrationally, to result in a surgeon becoming deskilled. This has been proved to be baseless, and the success of academic surgeons later on in their surgical careers is ample evidence to the contrary. A multi-institutional study on the psychological well-being of surgical trainees found that more than a third met the criteria for clinical psychological distress. This is significantly higher than that seen in societal controls.[6] Approaching deadlines and the lack of time has been shown to contribute largely to this.[5] Ability to overcome this is largely dependant on good time management and the ability to multitask where necessary. Achieving goals at the expense of mental and physical health defeats the objective of academic development and career progress. Striking a healthy balance between work, play and leisure should undoubtedly be the goal.

References

1. Souba WW, Gamelli RL, Lorber MI, Thompson JS, Kron IL, Hoyt DB. Strategies for success in academic surgery. *Surgery*. 1995; 117(1):90-5
2. Carrel T. The relationship between surgeon and the basic scientist. *Transpl Immunol*. 2002; 9(2-4):331-7
3. Seow CS, Teo NB, Wilson CR, Oien KA. Attitudes and training of research fellows in surgery; national questionnaire survey. *BMJ*. 2001;323(7315):725-726
4. Verrier ED. Getting started in academic cardiothoracic surgery. *J Thorac Cardiovasc Surg*. 2000;119(4 Pt 2):S1-10
5. Dutta S, Dunnington GL. Factors contributing to success in surgical education research. *Am J Surg*. 2000;179(3):247-9
6. Zare MS, Galanko J, Behrns KE, Koruda MJ, Boyle LM, Farley DR, Evens SRT, Meyer AA, Sheldon GF, Farrell TM. Psychological well-being of surgery residents before the 80-hour work week: a multiinstitutional study. *J Am Coll Surg*. 2004;198(4):634-40

Basic Science during Surgical Training

Viken Konyalian & Ravin R. Kumar

Historically, the academic surgeon has been committed to three major roles: patient care, research, and education. With the current health care environment in the United States and its increasing emphasis on clinical and administrative duties, dedication to basic science research has become increasingly difficult. This trend parallels changes in all medical specialties.[1] A review by Nahrwold et al.[2] showed that the number of articles devoted to basic and clinical research by American surgeons decreased from 1983 to 1993. Galt, similarly, showed a steady decline in publications by the members of the Society for Vascular Surgery during the 1990's.[3] Robert Conte noted this trend in his address to the Association for Academic Surgery, entitled "The Death of Academic Surgery?", citing a "greater dependence on clinical income to maintain academic viability," and urging for a resurgence in academic surgery.

The role of basic science research in a young surgeon's training has long been emphasized for multiple reasons. First, it provides an insight into pathophysiology, which eventually translates into improved understanding and outcome at the bedside. Late nineteenth century basic science investigations by the young neurosurgeon Cushing elucidated the relationship between increased intracranial pressure and respiratory drive. Carell highlighted similar examples of early basic science work that led to significant clinical advancements, including extra-corporeal perfusion and ischemia/

perfusion phenomena and their role in myocardial infarction, stroke, and shock.[4] Second, and perhaps of more importance to the surgical resident, the process of basic science investigation helps in the development of important problem-solving and reasoning skills. It requires the investigator to ask questions and create logical approaches to answering these questions. It also provides early exposure to the scientific method that involves formulation of a hypothesis, developing methodologies to test the hypothesis, analyzing data and publishing the result.

Multiple reviews have addressed the role, albeit changing, of basic science research in surgical training. Ko et al.[5] surveyed 85 senior-level academic surgeons regarding their basic science training and careers. 72% of respondents performed basic science research, and 71% attributed their research as a significant reason for choosing their subspecialty. 99% of those who performed basic science work during their training continued to do so after their training. 38% of those surveyed stopped research endeavors by age 39, and 17% at 40-49. Some of them cited increased clinical and administrative duties for the reduction in research activity.

Henke et al.[6] focused on basic science research and its role in postgraduate training, particularly vascular surgery training, elucidating the current trends. 74 Program directors and 259 fellows from vascular surgery programs approved by the Accreditation Council for Gradual Medical Education were surveyed. Among the fellows, 59% felt that research experience during general surgery residency helped secure a postgraduate position. A large proportion of program directors had similar research backgrounds. This study also highlights the current issues. Only one-third of programs offered a protected year of research, compared to 70% of programs in 1990. Most program directors emphasized clinical research during the fellowship, with less than half considering basic science work vital. The need for learning new clinical skills and technologies in exchange for dedicated research time explained this shift.

The attitudes of general surgery residents towards basic science research have generally been positive. In a large study involving 18 of the 20 general surgery training programs in New England, 450 surgical residents were surveyed.[7] Most of the residents surveyed planned to perform basic science research at some point of their training. 82% of those surveyed felt time spent in the lab provided a foundation for an academic career, while 83% felt their experience strengthened applications for fellowship. Work by Dunn et al.[8] reinforced this finding. They showed that half of surgical graduates that participated in research eventually held academic surgical positions, compared to only 13% of residents that did not participate in research.

Simultaneous surveys of surgical residents and their department chairs show diverging attitudes towards surgical research, although generally the perception is that a productive basic science laboratory experience is an important prerequisite for a successful career in academic surgery.[9] Chairpersons believe that the principal investigator's previous success was the major factor in residents decision about the laboratory in which to work. Residents place more value on their interest in the projects. The two groups also disagreed on who made the final decision regarding choice of the laboratory. Over 80% of the residents felt they made the decision, while chairpersons were evenly split between whether they or their residents made the choice. More chairpersons felt the major goal of the research experience was to learn reasoning and problem-solving skills, while more residents believed learning to write scientific publications was important.

Evolving pressures and trends in the surgical academic environment have muddled the criteria for promotion and advancement. Historically, research productivity has been the driving force behind promotion. Souba's survey of 101 chairpersons and academic surgeons cited publication record and research funding as the two most important factors for faculty promotion.[10] Presently, increased requirements for administrative, clinical, and instructive duties are difficult to quantify. Ambiguity in this regard has been attributed to some surgeons becoming disgruntled and leaving academia. Souba urged chairpersons to play an active role in reconciling this dilemma. He recommended establishing separate promotional tracks for surgeons focusing on research or clinical work. Surgeons with more clinical acumen would not necessarily engage in basic science research and vice versa.

Funding for all surgical academic endeavors, including basic science work, has become harder to attain. A survey of British academic surgeons revealed that over half had to self-fund attendance at academic meetings.[11] Only 20% of the research funding was provided by respective universities. Government funding supplied a small fraction of financial support for either research equipment or salaries.

Some academic surgeons have lobbied for a decreased emphasis on basic science research during surgical training, citing the previously mentioned increased responsibilities and stating that surgeons already suffer from "information overload." Most agree that the analytical skills developed with scientific investigation are valuable, but argue that alternative paths may teach these skills in a shorter time.[12]

In summary, the surgeon's time spent in a basic science laboratory can help hone problem-solving skills, while establishing a solid foundation for an academic career. Under the present conditions, dedicated time for such endeavors is becoming more and more difficult to achieve.

References

1. Brinkley WR. Disappearing physician-scientists. *Science*. 1999; 283: 291.
2. Nahrwold DL, Pereira SG, Dupuis J. United States research published in major surgical journals is decreasing. *Ann Surg*. 1995; 222 (3): 263-6.
3. Galt SW, Kraiss LW, Sarfati MR. Has the changing nature of vascular surgery adversely affected scholarly activity? *J Vasc Surg*. 2003; 38: 1-6.
4. Carrel, T. The relationship between surgeon and basic scientist. *Transplant Immunology*. 2002; 9: 331-337.
5. Ko CY, Whang EE, Longmire WP Jr, McFadden DW. Improving the surgeon's participation in research: is it a problem of training or priority? *J Surg Res*. 2000; 91: 5-8.
6. Henke PK, Kish P, Stanley JC. Relevance of basic laboratory and clinical research activities as part of the vascular surgery fellowship: an assessment by program directors and postfellowship surgeons. *J Vasc Surg*. 2002; 36: 1083-91.
7. Stewart RD, Doyle J, Lollis SS, Stone MD. Surgical resident research in New England. *Arch Surg*. 2000; 135: 439-44.
8. Dunn JC, Lai EC, Brooks CM, Stabile BE, Fonkalsrud EW. The outcome of research training during surgical residency. *J Pediatr Surg*. 1998; 33: 362-4.
9. Souba WW, Tanabe KK, Gadd MA, Smith BL, Bushman MS. Attitudes and opinions toward surgical research: a survey of surgical residents and their chairpersons. *Annals of Surgery*. 1996; 223: 377-383.

10. Souba WW, Gamelli RL, Lorber MI, Thompson JS, Kron IL, Tompkins RG, Hoyt DB. Strategies for success in academic surgery. *Surgery*. 1995; 117: 90-5.
11. Davies AH, Locke-Edmunds JC, Magee TR, Farndon JR. The cost, funding and acceptance of surgical research. *Ann R Coll Surg Engl*. 1994; 76: 185-6.
12. Pietroni, MC. Surgical training and research. *Ann R Coll Surg Engl*. 1994; 76: 115-116.

Writing a Research Protocol for Studies Involving Human Subjects

Christine Dauphine & Christian De Virgilio

A research protocol is a document which states specific conditions for the conduction of a given research project. It is like a contract between the investigator, the research community, the human subjects and the institutional review board. Once the conditions are agreed upon, research is to be conducted exactly according to the protocol and all deviations from it must be amended to the protocol in advance. The research protocol is official documentation of specifically what is to be done in a given project. It is the means to obtaining approval from the ethical, peer and administrative review boards. It is also the manual according to which investigational team members and aids will uniformly carry out the study design.

Why is a Research Protocol Necessary?

Sixty years ago, the Nazi Germans were able to perform humiliating, painful mutilations on prisoners of concentration camps under the disguise of "scientific research." Around the same time, in the United States, poor black men with syphilis were deliberately not treated despite the availability of penicillin in order to study the disease.[1] The U.S. Government also sponsored thousands of human radiation experiments from 1944 to 1974 that were carried out without consent in most cases, and sometimes in children and prisoners.[1] Lack of ethical research methods and reports of outright harm to study subjects began to jeopardize the public's trust and willingness to participate in research. This amounts to a lack of trust by the public of researchers, in general. The research community is thus judged by how it conducts research.

Over the years, federal laws and review boards have been established to guarantee protection of human subjects and to ensure that research is purposeful, beneficial and not harmful to study participants. After the Second World War, and, as a part of the settlement of the Nuremburg Trials, The Nuremberg Code of Ethics in Medical Research was created to regulate research using human subjects, setting moral standards for research and initiating the idea of an institutional review committee.[1-3] In 1964, The Eighteenth World Assembly adopted The World Medical Association Declaration of Helsinki, which produced a set of recommendations in order to guide investigators planning biomedical research with human subjects. This Declaration has undergone five revisions since its inception.[1, 2, 4, 5]

In 1974, the United States Congress passed the National Research Act, which mandated the formation of the National Commission for the Protection of Human Subjects of Biomedical and Behavioral Research.[5] In 1979, this commission produced a report entitled Ethical Principles and Guidelines for the Protection of Human Subjects of Research.[4,5] More popularly known as the Belmont Report, this document describes three basic principles of ethics that are to guide the decisions to be made by institutional review boards regarding research involving human subjects. Briefly, the first principle is Respect for Persons, where individuals are seen as autonomous and must be given complete information in terms that they can understand in order to give voluntary consent to participate or withdraw from a study. Second is the principle of Beneficence, which focuses on the balance between ensuring that individuals are not harmed and the importance of the research to the overall advancement of medicine and necessity for knowledge in that area. Justice, the third principle, is to be considered when selecting patients for the study, distributing burdens and benefits equally among participants. For example, subjects should be members of the group most likely to benefit from the research, risks should not be placed unduly on subjects that are unlikely to benefit from the results, and groups, such as children and pregnant women, should not be excluded from projects from which they may benefit. These three principles are the basis for all federal regulations that govern research on human subjects.

Many other countries are beginning to follow the U.S. model for regulating research.[3, 6] However, some developing countries still lack effective ethics review committees, where research subjects are still subjected to undue risks not disclosed to them during a consent process.[7] The establishment of these ethics review committees was recently the focus of the 2nd Symposium on Ethical Issues in Health Research in Developing Countries held in Pakistan in August 2003.[7]

The research community is now held responsible for its scientific endeavors, to conduct ethical research. Human subjects have right to informed consent and privacy, which must be upheld at all times, and research must not be deceptive, pain-invoking, injurious or humiliating. A research protocol must embody all of the above principles and show compliance to federal regulations. Therefore, the research protocol is pivotal to the conduct of research at an institution, as it provides a common understanding of what is to be done to human subjects, and specifically states compliance to the regulations that protect human subjects.

Who Approves the Research Protocol?

In most large institutions, there are three separate components of the review and approval of a research protocol. The first is a peer review, which is sometimes referred to as a Medical Review Board or Scientific Review Board, whose aim is to ensure that the research objectives and methods are meritorious.[2, 8] This committee is typically composed of scientist or physician experts in the general area of science or medicine that is to be researched. Their goal is to ascertain that the anticipated conclusions can reasonably be reached using the proposed methods, and that the knowledge gained by the study is useful and worth carrying out the study. The second component is an administrative review of grants and contracts that exist between the investigator, the institution, and the sponsors of the research project. This committee's primary purpose is to outline or dictate who owns the data, who is responsible for injuries to subjects, what outside institutions or sponsors are part of the study, and who may have financial or other interests that directly impact the study design and conclusions. Finally, and perhaps most crucial, is the execution of an ethical review to ensure that research does not violate the rights or welfare of human subjects. At most institutions this is referred to as the Institutional Review Board (IRB).

What is an Institutional Review Board (IRB) and What is its Role?

All institutions at which research is at least partly government-sponsored are mandated to file an Assurance of Compliance with the federal government, agreeing to comply with federal regulations regarding research and the protection of human subjects.[1, 4] These assurances are overseen by the federal Office for Protection from Research Risk (OPRR), and apply to all research that is carried out by the institution, regardless of government sponsorship. Under this assurance, the institution is required to establish an Institutional Review Board (IRB) in order to ensure that all projects are in compliance with federal regulations. The IRB is a multidisciplinary committee, composed of physicians, nurses, ethicists, pharmacists, social workers, and clergy, and its performance is overseen by the OPRR.[2,8] The IRB is responsible for approving research protocols, paying specific attention to the balance between obtaining clinically important data and the risks imposed upon human subjects. Ideally, results of the study will contribute greatly to the advances of medicine, while minimizing risks and avoiding harm to the participants. The IRB oversees the consent process, ensuring that subjects are fully informed of risks and benefits they may reasonably expect by participation in the study. The board must also routinely monitor all research at the institution; suspend projects that are not in compliance with the protocol or regulations of the IRB, and report to the federal government any on-going noncompliance with regulations or injury to subjects. This ensures that the rights and safety of human subjects are not compromised, that adequately trained staff manage the study, that the study is carefully documented, and, finally, that the protocol is strictly adhered to. In the past year, it has been recommended that ethics review boards also be held responsible for enforcing public dissemination of results of research.[9]

Writing a Research Protocol

Exact forms and processes will be unique to every institution, but, in general, the protocol will embody the following information.

1. **Objective**. An overall objective of the research, outlining the aims of the research project.
2. **Background information**. Background information, outlining other recent significant research conclusions relating to the specific area of study. Specifically to be noted are the results of research previously performed in animal experiments.
3. **Research methods**. Description of research methods, including the rationale behind the chosen approach and descriptions of all experimental procedures. Specifically outline what is to be done to human subjects. If surveys, questionnaires, or forms for data collection are to be used, these should also be attached and submitted with the protocol. Methods regarding confidentiality should also be stated.
4. **Data analysis/statistics**. Include an anticipation and justification for the number of study subjects. Explain procedures for data monitoring and statistical analysis. Also, disclose who is to perform data analysis, who is responsible for the reporting of all results, and what is the relation of these persons to the investigator.
5. **Summary**. A brief summary written in lay terms, outlining the above components of the protocol. This summary is intended for the persons on the ethics committee who do not have an extensive scientific or medical background.

How to Address Issues Regarding Human Subjects

Most institutions will require a separate section of the protocol to address issues pertaining to human subjects. This may exist in many formats, but, overall, incorporates the following issues:

1. **Inclusion/exclusion criteria**. State, in specific terms, who the study subjects are going to be, including descriptions of age, race, and sex distributions. Justify the use or non-use of minorities, children, mentally incapacitated patients, pregnant women or foreign language speakers. Explain how the data expected to be gleaned

from the study will be applicable to the population as a whole. Specifically, be sure to describe how the chosen study group, which is to bear the burden of risk, is representative of the group most likely to benefit from the results of the project.

2. **Potential risks**. Delineate all potential risks to the study subjects, and predict the likelihood of occurrence of each. Risks can be physical, psychological, social, legal or financial in nature. Use supportive data from previous experience in international studies or animal research. State all precautions that will be taken to minimize risks. For protocols involving potential for life-threatening reactions, list all precautionary measures that will be taken, all resuscitative equipment that will be made available, and the availability of emergency medical support at the location where research is performed and during the hours of operation.[10]

3. **Potential benefits**. Describe all potential benefits that can reasonably be expected for the individual as well as for society. Include potential therapeutic benefits that may be expected for participants. Make a statement regarding the importance of the study results, and how this outweighs the potential risks to the subjects.

4. **Non-participants**. State all risks and benefits that can reasonably be expected for an individual who declines to participate, or who withdraws from the project at anytime during the study.

5. **Recruitment of subjects**. Give a list of planned approaches to recruiting patients to the study. Examples include flyers, contact letters, media, and physician referrals. Describe who will be explaining the study to the patients. This person must be knowledgeable regarding specific risks/benefits to each participant, and should initially be someone other than the primary investigator.[2] Disclose any referral fees that will be paid to physicians and/or patients.[3]

6. **Vulnerable subjects**. Prisoners, economically disadvantaged persons, critically ill patients, cancer victims, children and the mentally disabled are examples of vulnerable subjects. These groups may not be able to understand the risks of participating in research or may be desperate enough to overlook significant risks in order to potentially gain. The treatment of these groups must be described, with special attention to how they are recruited and informed.

7. **Studies requiring deception**. Often, subjects of a study need to be deceived in order to scientifically test a drug or method.

The use of a placebo is an example of deception. If this is required, state why the project could not otherwise be done without deceiving subjects. Describe specific procedures planned for "debriefing" subjects when the study is over. State by whom and how subjects will be told of this deception.

8. **Costs and reimbursements**. Disclose all anticipated costs and reimbursements to study subjects. If multiple patient contacts are required, state who is to pay for these visits, and how long direct contact will be required. If the patient is to suffer a complication as a result of the experiment, state who will be responsible for the cost to the patient.

9. **Privacy**. Explain all procedures for ensuring security of research data and maintaining patient confidentiality. This includes how data will be recorded, where it will be stored, who will have access to it, and how will it be destroyed when no longer necessary.

Writing a Consent Document

After an in-depth explanation of the purpose, risks, and benefits of the research project, the subject's signature must be obtained on a written consent form, documenting his/her understanding of the conversation. The form must be written in language that is comprehensible to the participant, using terms that do not extend past the level of high school education. Consent should still be obtained from children and mentally incapacitated individuals, but permission to participate must be granted by the patient's guardian. The Department of Health and Human Services established the following eight guidelines for writing a document of informed consent[4, 11]:

1. A statement that the study involves research, an explanation of the purposes of the research, and the expected duration of the subject's participation, a description of the procedures to be followed, and identification of any procedures which are experimental;

2. A description of any reasonably foreseeable risks or discomforts to the subject;

3. A description of any benefits to the subject or to others which may reasonably be expected from the research;

4. A disclosure of appropriate alternative procedures of courses of treatment, if any, that might be advantageous to the subject;

5. A statement describing the extent, if any, to which confidentiality of records identifying the subject will be maintained;

6. For research involving more than minimal risk, an explanation as to whether any compensation or any medical treatments are available if injury occurs and, if so, what they consist of or where further information may be obtained;

7. An explanation of whom to contact for answers to pertinent questions about the research and research subject's rights and whom to contact in the event of a research-related injury to the subject, and;

8. A statement that participation is voluntary, refusal to participate will involve no penalty or loss of benefits to which the subject is otherwise entitled, and that the subject may discontinue participation at any time without penalty or loss of benefits to which the subject is otherwise entitled.

What about Research not Directly Involving Human Subjects?

Research projects which involve chart reviews and retrospective data collection often do not involve the study subjects directly. There is no patient contact, and the risk to the individual is considered minimal, often pertaining only to confidentiality issues. For this research, an expedited review is possible, where approval of a project may be obtained directly from the director or chair of the IRB, without review by the entire committee. A research protocol is still necessary, and should address all of the previously discussed issues, including a justification for minimal risk to the study participants. It is recommended that the case be discussed briefly with a representative of the IRB to determine whether a project qualifies for this type of review to avoid wasting precious time, having the proposal later requested for full review.

Comments

Of course, review boards and procedures will be slightly different at individual institutions, and interpretations of regulations are dependent upon the members who comprise each board. So, researchers should always contact the IRB at their institution prior to embarking on writing a protocol in order to obtain the necessary forms and inquire about specific procedures. If an unusual circumstance regarding human subjects exists, consulting first with a member of the IRB is recommended. In a study on IRB responses to submitted proposals, it was found that only 24% were approved without request for further information or changes to the protocol.[12] Be prepared; the entire process can take weeks to months before an approval to proceed with the project is issued.

References

1. Dunn C, Chadwick G. *Protecting Study Volunteers in Research.* Boston: CenterWatch, Inc; 1999.
2. Kamienski M. Tips on navigating your research proposal through the institutional review board. *J Emerg Nurs.* 2000;26(2):178-81.
3. Fiscus PW. Protecting human research subjects. *J Biolaw Bus.* 2001;4(4):18-22.
4. United States regulatory requirements for research involving human subjects. *J Biolaw Bus.* 1998;1(2):39-53.
5. Knudson, PL. Ethical principles in human subject research. *Arch Med Res.* 2001;32(5):473-4.
6. Allen PA, Waters WE. Development of an ethical committee and its effect on research design. *Lancet.* 1982;1(8283):1233-6.
7. Ahmad, K. Developing countries need effective ethics review committees. *Lancet.* 2003;362(9384):627.
8. Drazen, JM. Controlling Research Trials. *N Engl J Med.* 2003;348(14):1377-80.
9. Mann, H. Research ethics committees and public dissemination of clinical trial results. *Lancet.* 2002;360:406-8.
10. Hamilos DL, Oppenheimer JJ, Nelson HS. Suggested approaches for research protocols involving the potential for life-threatening reactions. *J Allergy Clin Immunol.* 1993;91(6):1101-20.
11. Nokes, KM. Exploring the Institutional Review Board Process. *J N Y State Nurses Assoc.* 1989;20(3):7-10.
12. Kent G. Responses by four Local Research Ethics Committees to submitted proposals. *J Med Ethics.* 1999;25:274-7.

Introduction to Statistics for Surgical Research

Jason S. Haukoos

Introduction

Research is a process. Although this chapter focuses on statistical analysis, it is important to remember the fundamental tenets of performing clinical research. These include developing an appropriate question, designing study to effectively answer the question, implementing the study in an efficient and effective manner, and collecting and assimilating the data. Use of appropriate methods for collecting, assimilating, and storing data cannot be over-emphasized. No statistical algorithm or technique will make up for a poorly designed study, or poorly acquired data. It is important to plan all elements of the study, including how data will be collected and stored, and what types of analyses will be performed, prior to beginning of the project.

      The goals of this chapter are to introduce the reader to basic and advanced statistical concepts, including: (1) data collection and storage; (2) the concepts of populations, samples, and distributions; (3) descriptive statistics; (4) inferential statistics; and (5) sample size determination. It is not the goal of this chapter to describe in full detail how to perform these analyses. There are many existing textbooks that do this nicely. Instead, most of what is written in this chapter is a conceptual framework for thinking about analyses, with emphasis on their utility and when to perform them.

Data Collection and Representation

Almost uniformly, data are collected and assimilated into an r × c table, where r represents rows and c represents columns. This two-dimensional representation of data includes a specific number of observations (r) and variables (c), depending on the study. In most instances in clinical research, an observation will represent a patient or patient encounter, and multiple variables (or characteristics) that vary from one observation to another will be collected. It is important for the researcher to define the variables that will be collected prior to initiating the study. Once this is done, data are collected through a study-specific data collection process, and are then entered into a database (Table 5.1). Once the database is complete, descriptive and inferential statistical analyses are performed. Several software packages are available to perform these analyses.

Table 5.1. Database example [Each row corresponds to an observation and each column corresponds to a specific variable.]

	Variables			
Observations	Age	Sex	Heart Rate	Survival
Patient #1	35	M	120	Yes
Patient #2	45	F	100	Yes
Patient #3	25	F	90	No
Patient #4	50	M	80	No
.	.	.	.	.
.	.	.	.	.
.	.	.	.	.
Patient #500	33	F	110	Yes

Populations, Samples and Distributions

It is important to understand and distinguish between populations and samples. A *population* is defined generally as all individuals in a group and is often referred to as the *base population*. It is this cohort, or group of subjects, that investigators attempt to draw conclusions about. Unfortunately, this group is rarely studied in its entirety. Instead, investigators sample from the base population (this sample is called the *study population*). The study population is a subset of, and is used to draw conclusions about, the base population. As an example, a base population may include all patients with ruptured abdominal aortic aneurysms (AAAs). Of course, if you wanted to study patients with ruptured AAAs, it would be impractical (and impossible) to study all ruptured AAA patients. Instead, you would sample from this population, perform analyses on the sample, and draw conclusions about the base population.

Several measures help to characterize a population. We estimate population parameters (or measures that describe a population) by calculating statistics from the study population. For instance, we may calculate a mean from the study population in order to describe the center of a specific variable (e.g. the size of AAAs), and this will act as an estimate for the base population.

Frequency distributions are defined as the total number of observations among all possible categories for a specific variable, and are represented either in tabular or graphical formats. The two most common frequency distributions are the bell-shaped distribution and the skewed distribution. A bell-shaped distribution, often referred to as a normal or Gaussian distribution, is a symmetric bell-shaped curve, whereas a skewed distribution is an asymmetric curve in which more data elements are grouped to one side of the distribution range (Figs 5.1 and 5.2). Differentiating between these two fundamental types of frequency distributions is important as it dictates how data should be represented and what types of statistical analyses need to be performed. A *probability distribution* should not be confused with a frequency distribution. A probability distribution is a curve

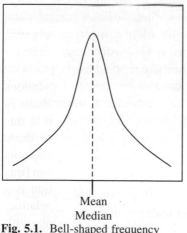

Mean
Median

Fig. 5.1. Bell-shaped frequency distribution

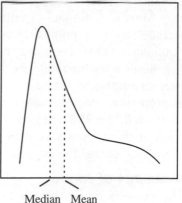

Median Mean

Fig. 5.2. Skewed frequency distribution

that shows all the values that a variable can take and the likelihood that each will occur, and is defined mathematically. Examples of some common probability distributions include the normal, binomial, logit, and Poisson distributions.

Descriptive Statistics

The first step in representing data includes reporting summary (also known as descriptive or univariate) statistics. Descriptive statistics are one of the most fundamental ways to represent data and are used to organize and summarize groups of observations. It is impractical for the researcher to report all raw data elements (i.e. the actual data), and, therefore, an attempt to summarize such data must be made.

Types of data

Data can be represented in several different ways and it is important to understand their basic structures. Data may be represented as numbers (e.g. 0.1, 1, 2, etc.) or as characters (e.g. Yes or No, Male or Female); and numerical data can be converted to character data, and vice versa (e.g. 1=Male and 2=Female). Numerical data are generally divided into either continuous or discrete categories. *Continuous data* are defined as data that represent measurable quantities that are not restricted to specific values. Common examples of continuous variables are age and temperature. *Discrete*, or *categorical*, *data* are defined as measurable quantities that are restricted to specific values. Common examples of categorical variables are sex and race/ethnicity.

Most descriptions of either continuous or categorical data include reporting point estimates with their respective spreads. Continuous data are commonly reported as values of central tendency (e.g. mean or median) and their variability (e.g. standard deviation or inter-quartile range), whereas categorical data are commonly reported as proportions or percentages with 95% confidence intervals (e.g. 25/100 = 0.25 = 25% and its 95% confidence interval: 17% to 35%). Each of these reports an estimate with a degree of variation or confidence around the estimate.

Measures of centre

The *mean* is the arithmetic average of the data, and, although commonly reported, is the most valid measure of center only when the data are normally distributed. However, most clinical data are *not* distributed normally. Instead, most data collected in a clinical environment have skewed frequency distributions. When data have a skewed frequency distribution, the *median*, or the value that represents the 50th percentile, should be reported. The 50th percentile represents the middle measurement in an ordered set of data, and is a more valid measure of center when the frequency distribution is skewed because the mean is more vulnerable to outliers, or extreme values (i.e. values that contribute to the longer tail of a skewed frequency distribution) (Fig. 5.2). The *mode*, which represents the most common value, is generally not reported in clinical research.

Measures of dispersion or variability

Measures of center act as point estimates and do not describe variation around the estimate. Instead, variability is generally represented as ranges, standard deviations (SD), standard error of the mean (SEM), inter-quartile ranges, or confidence intervals. Each of these is reported differently, depending on what the investigator is trying to convey.

The range is the most simple variability measure and is defined by the two most extreme values for a particular variable. Unfortunately, the range is influenced significantly by outlying data points, thus limiting its usefulness.

Standard deviation is calculated from another measure of variability called the variance. The variance is a measure of the deviation of each data point from the calculated mean for that particular variable. These measures are squared, summed, and then divided by the number of observations (n) minus 1. The variance represents, in general, the variation from the mean, and the SD is simply the square root of the variance. The SD is generally reported with the mean.

Standard error of the mean equals the standard deviation divided by the square root of the number of observations in the dataset. By this, it is easy to see that the SEM will always be smaller than the SD. The SEM is most commonly used to calculate confidence intervals (see below), and should not be confused with, or used in place of, the SD. Standard deviation is a valid measure of variation around the mean, whereas SEM is not.

The *inter-quartile range* (IQR) is represented by the 25th and 75th percentiles, and is generally reported with the median. The 25th percentile represents the measurement in which one-fourth of all ranked observations for a particular variable are smaller, whereas the

75th percentile represents the measurement in which three-fourths of all ranked observations for a particular variable are smaller. When the frequency distribution of a particular variable is skewed, the median and IQR are more valid measures of center and dispersion than the mean and SD.

Confidence intervals represent a range of values likely to be representative of the population parameter (i.e. the parameter from the base population) that was estimated from the study population. For example, the 95% confidence interval around a mean implies that if the study was repeated 100 times, in 95 of the studies, the true population parameter would fall within the 95% confidence interval. The confidence interval relies on the variability of the data as well as the size of the sample (i.e. SEM). There are several formulas for estimating confidence intervals, and there are several excellent references that describe this process in detail.

Epidemiological measures

Several other research-related terms deserve defining and clarification. Investigators frequently misuse terms such as rates, ratios, risks, incidence, and prevalence. There are three fundamental types of mathematical quantities that are used to summarize categorical, or discrete, data, also known as basic epidemiological measures. These include proportions, ratios, and rates. A *proportion* is a fraction in which all elements of the numerator are included in the denominator. Proportions are unit-less and their values range from 0 to 1 (e.g. 25/100 = 0.25). You may also multiply proportions by 100 to express them as *percentages*. A *ratio* is another type of fraction in which elements of the numerator are not necessarily included in the denominator. An example of this includes a ratio of two proportions, like the likelihood ratio. A *rate* is another type of fraction, which reflects the instantaneous change in one quantity per unit change in another quantity (the denominator is usually time related). Unlike proportions, rates have units and are not bound by 1 (e.g. cases per year).

Risk is an incidence measure that defines the probability of developing the disease during a given period or time interval. Risk is a proportion that requires a time reference. For example, a 3% risk of death over 3 months is different from a 3% risk of death over 30 years.

Adding another level to basic epidemiological measures, we define the incidence and prevalence, both of which are types of frequency measures. With *incidence*, the numerator reflects the number of new cases identified during a given time period, whereas with *prevalence*, the numerator reflects the number of existing cases at a specific time during a given time period.

Inferential Statistics

In a general sense, statistical inference refers to the use of statistics for deriving inferences about your data. Specifically, statistical inference involves the testing of hypotheses, and is also known as significance or classical statistical testing. Hypotheses are numerical statements about population parameters and are generally stated in terms of a null hypothesis (H_0) and an alternative hypothesis (H_1). In general, the null hypothesis makes a statement about no effect, whereas the alternative hypothesis makes a statement about an effect. For example, a null hypothesis in the context of the effectiveness of two specific vasopressors A and B in the setting of distributive shock might state that there is no difference in survival (the outcome) when vasopressor A is used in comparison to vasopressor B. On the other hand, the alternative hypothesis might state that there is a difference in survival when vasopressor A is used in comparison to vasopressor B. Using statistical testing, we either reject or fail to reject (i.e. accept) the null hypothesis. Statistical testing always centers on the null hypothesis because the null hypothesis is strictly defined, whereas the alternative hypothesis can assume an infinite number of possibilities. As with the example above, the null hypothesis states that there is no effect. However, the alternative hypothesis states that there is an effect, but does not specifically indicate the magnitude or direction of that effect.

Two types of errors can occur when performing classical statistical testing, namely, type I and type II errors. A *type I error* is defined as rejecting the null hypothesis when in fact it is true. In essence, an effect is found when really there is not one, and the probability of committing a type I error is referred to as alpha (α). A *type II error* is defined as not rejecting (i.e. accepting) the null hypothesis when in fact it is false. In essence, not finding an effect when one actually exists, and the probability of committing a type II error is referred to as beta (β). *Power* is defined as $1 - \beta$, or the probability of rejecting the null hypothesis when it is false. In essence, finding an effect when one actually exists (Fig. 5.3).

Truth in the Population

		Association	No Association
Results in the Study Sample	**Reject** H_0	Power	Type I error
	Fail to Reject H_0	Type II error	Correct

Fig. 5.3. 2 × 2 table representing the four possible significance testing outcomes

Medical literature is wrought with references to "statistical significance", as reported by p-values. The *p-value* is a continuous measure (a probability ranging from 0 to 1) of the compatibility between the hypothesis and the data. Thus, as the p-value approaches zero, the probability of rejecting the null hypothesis increases, whereas as the p-value approaches one, the probability of rejecting the null hypothesis decreases. The p-value is calculated from the data using various statistical tests. The distinction between significance and non-significance is, however, arbitrary and must be used with caution. In the most classic sense, p-values ≤0.05 are considered "significant".

The *alpha level* (α) is a fixed point (usually set to 0.05), which represents the probability of committing a type I error. Unfortunately, the distinction between the p-value and α is blurred, even among some statisticians. It is important not to interpret the p-value as the alpha level for a particular hypothesis test, and thus the p-value is not the probability of committing a type I error for a particular test. Instead, the p-value is the probability of obtaining the results observed, or results more inconsistent with the null hypothesis, given that the null hypothesis is true. From a practical perspective, it is absurd to consider a p-value = 0.06 not significant, but to consider a p-value = 0.05 significant.

There are several limitations to reporting p-values, all of which can be remedied by reporting confidence intervals. The confidence interval is directly related to the p-value. If the 95% confidence interval includes the null value (e.g. zero as a measure of difference or 1 for an odds ratio), then the corresponding p-value will be > 0.05, if the lower limit of the 95% confidence interval equals zero exactly, then the corresponding p-value will equal 0.05 exactly, and if the 95% confidence interval excludes zero, then the corresponding p-value will be < 0.05. Confidence intervals in this manner convey not only "statistical significance", but also the certainty of the effect (as represented by the width of the confidence interval), and the magnitude of effect. In addition, if the confidence interval includes zero (i.e. the difference is not considered "statistically significant"), it will also suggest whether the effect is truly not significant or whether there were not enough patients in the study to reliably detect a clinically-important difference, if it really existed.

Measures of validity

Sensitivity, specificity, and predictive values are commonly used to assess the validity of diagnostic tests. In order to calculate these measures, the diagnostic test needs to be compared with the "gold standard" for making the specific diagnosis. Consider the following example. An investigator wants to test a new biomarker obtained from patients' serum for detecting colorectal carcinoma. If this biomarker is present, then colorectal carcinoma is presumed to be present, whereas if it is not present, then it is presumed that the patient is free from the disease. The investigator identifies 100 total patients, 30 of whom have biopsy-proven colorectal carcinoma, and 70 of whom do not. He obtains blood from each patient and tests the serum for this particular biomarker. Of the 100 patients, 20 test positive for the biomarker, whereas 80 do not, and in 18 cases, the biomarker is present and the patient was diagnosed with colorectal carcinoma. These data can be placed into a 2 × 2 table to assist in assessing validity (Fig. 5.4).

Sensitivity is defined as the proportion of those with the condition who have a positive test, and is calculated, in general, as a/(a+c). *Specificity* is defined as the proportion of those without the condition who have a negative test, and is calculated, in general, as d/(b+d). The *positive predictive value* (PPV) is defined as the proportion of those with a positive test who have the condition, and is calculated, in general, as a/(a+b). The *negative predictive value* (NPV) is defined as the proportion of those with negative test who do not have the condition, and is calculated, in general, as d/(c+d). When reporting measures of validity, as with all proportions, confidence intervals should be reported.

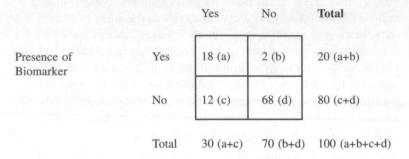

Biopsy-Proven Disease

		Yes	No	**Total**
Presence of Biomarker	Yes	18 (a)	2 (b)	20 (a+b)
	No	12 (c)	68 (d)	80 (c+d)
	Total	30 (a+c)	70 (b+d)	100 (a+b+c+d)

Sensitivity = 18/30 = 60% (95% CI: 41% - 77%)
Specificity = 68/70 = 97% (95% CI: 90% - 100%)
PPV = 18/20 = 90% (95% CI: 68% - 99%)
NPV = 68/80 = 85% (95% CI: 75% - 92%)

Fig.5.4. 2 × 2 table to assess the utility of a biomarker in diagnosing colorectal carcinoma (Positive predictive value = PPV and negative predictive value = NPV)

Sensitivity and specificity are not affected by the prevalence of disease within the population, whereas PPV and NPV are affected by the prevalence of disease within the population. The PPV will decrease while the NPV will increase as the prevalence of disease in the population decreases.

Introduction to Statistical Techniques

The term "univariate" refers to a type of analysis involving a single variable and is synonymous with descriptive statistics. The term "bivariate" refers to a type of analysis that tests the association between two variables, and specific statistical tests are used to test this association. Finally, the term "multivariate" refers to a type of analysis that tests associations between more than two variables.

Bivariate statistical techniques

There are many commonly used statistical techniques for assessing bivariate relationships. The most fundamental and commonly used techniques can be divided into parametric and non-parametric tests. Parametric tests assume that the structures of the variables conform to a specific probability distribution, whereas non-parametric tests do not hold such distributional assumptions.

Student's t test is parametric and compares the means of two groups. Its principal assumptions are that the variable is continuous and normally distributed with equal variances. Its non-parametric counterpart is the *Wilcoxon rank sum test* (also known as the *Mann Whitney U test*), which compares the medians of two groups. This statistical test only requires the variable to be continuous. *One-way analysis of variance* (ANOVA) requires the same assumptions as Student's t test; however, it compares the means across three or more groups. Its non-parametric counterpart is the *Kruskal-Wallis test*, which compares the medians of three or more groups.

The *chi-square test* compares proportions between two or more groups and its principal assumption is that there are ≥ 5 expected counts in all cells of the 2×2 table. *Fisher's exact test* also compares proportions between two or more groups, but does not require ≥ 5 expected counts in all cells.

Tests of agreement are other forms of bivariate analyses. These statistical tests are classified into two broad groups, those that compare continuous variables and those that compare categorical variables. The *Pearson correlation coefficient* is a parametric test that tests correlation between two continuous variables, and the *Spearman rank correlation coefficient* is its non-parametric counterpart. If the variables are categorical, then *Cohen's kappa* is used to determine the level of agreement.

Multiple comparisons

Multiple comparisons refer to performing multiple independent statistical tests and drawing conclusions from the reported p-values. Unfortunately, the investigator increases the risk of making a type I error (i.e. rejecting the null hypothesis when in fact it is true, or finding a difference when one does not exist) as the number of statistical tests increases. This can be corrected by performing a *Bonferroni correction*, which corrects the alpha (usually designated at 0.05) by dividing it by the number of statistical tests that will be performed. For example, if 5 tests are planned, then the adjusted alpha will equal 0.01 (0.05/5).

Multivariate statistical techniques

There are many types of multivariate statistical techniques, including both parametric and non-parametric forms. The most recognized techniques are parametric regression techniques, and include multivariate, or multiple, linear regression and logistic regression. *Linear regression* refers to the dependent variable being continuous, whereas *logistic regression* refers to the dependent variable being binary categorical. The fundamental structure of these models is the same. Independent variables (also known as predictor or explanatory variables) are placed into the model, and are used to "predict" or "explain" a single dependent variable (also known as an outcome variable). The goal is to assess the effect of one independent variable on the dependent variable while controlling for other, potentially confounding, independent variables. From an epidemiological perspective, *confounders* are loosely defined as variables that are associated with an explanatory variable and the outcome variable (Fig. 5.5). If only one variable is used as the independent variable, then the analysis becomes bivariate.

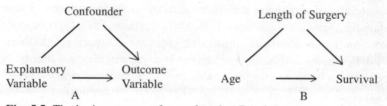

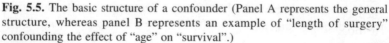

Fig. 5.5. The basic structure of a confounder (Panel A represents the general structure, whereas panel B represents an example of "length of surgery" confounding the effect of "age" on "survival".)

For example, an investigator may want to assess the effect of a patient's age on survival in patients who undergo coronary artery bypass surgery (CABG). The investigator collects data from 500 patients who underwent CABG. Data were collected for survival to hospital discharge (Yes or No), the age of each patient (as a continuous variable), and potential confounders, including the length of the surgery (in minutes), comorbidities, cardiac ejection fraction prior to surgery, and the number of bypass grafts required.

It is possible, even probable, that if separate bivariate analyses were performed for age and survival and length of surgery and survival, both would demonstrate statistical associations, independent of each other. However, it is possible that age is not associated with survival after controlling (or adjusting) for the length of surgery. By introducing both independent variables into the same logistic regression model, you are able to determine the effect of age on survival, adjusted for the length of the procedure.

Survival analysis

Survival analysis incorporates the same general structure of bivariate and multivariate statistical analyses, with one exception. The measurement scale of the outcome variable is different. For instance, the outcome variable for linear analyses is continuous and the outcome variable for logistic analyses is binary categorical. With survival data, the outcome variable is time-dependent and can be classified as any unit of time (e.g. seconds, minutes, days, years, etc.).

The bivariate form of survival analysis is represented by survival curves (also known as *Kaplan-Meier curves*), and the test that assesses for a statistical difference between the curves is called the *log rank test*. The multivariate form of survival analysis is called the *Cox proportional hazard regression* and holds the same form as all multivariate analyses, except for the structure of the dependent, or outcome, variable, which is again time-dependent.

Sample Size Determination

Sample size calculations (also known as power calculations) are generally viewed as calculations to determine the number of subjects needed for a particular study to show statistical significance. Under a more specific framework, sample size calculations are used to determine the number of subjects needed for a particular study in order to reject the null hypothesis using a specific statistical test. Although this section is placed towards the end of this chapter, it is paramount to perform the sample size calculation prior to initiating the study.

In order to perform a sample size calculation, the investigator must specify, *a priori*, alpha (the probability of a type I error), beta (the probability of a type II error), the minimum magnitude of effect that is regarded as important to detect, and the expected frequency of disease or exposure. Several computer programs are available for doing a wide variety of sample size calculations.

Conclusions

Statistical theory is extraordinarily deep, and it is easy to get confused by specific terminology and methods involved in performing analyses.

In addition, over the past decade, research methodologies and statistical techniques have become more sophisticated. However, the basic tenet of statistical analysis is to provide means to derive inferences from data. It is important to have a fundamental understanding of basic statistical techniques, and to seek out statistical expertise prior to performing, and during, a study.

Acknowledgement

I am grateful to Stephen Wall, MD, MPH and Stephen Wolf, MD for sharing their individual perspectives and helpful suggestions during the preparation of this chapter.

References

1.   Rothman KJ, Greenland S. *Modern Epidemiology.* 2nd ed. New York: Lippincott Williams & Wilkins, 1998.
2.   Zar JH. *Biostatistical Analysis.* 4th ed. New Jersey: Prentice Hall, 1999.
3.   Pagano M, Gauvreau K. *Principles of Biostatistics.* California: Duxbury Press, 1993.
4.   Agresti A. *Categorical Data Analysis.* 2nd ed. New Jersey: John Wiley & Sons, Inc., 2002.
5.   Hosmer DW, Lemeshow S. *Applied Logistic Regression.* 2nd ed. New York: John Wiley & Sons, Inc., 2000.
6.   Hosmer DW, Lemeshow S. *Applied Survival Analysis: Regression Modeling of Time to Event Data.* New York: John Wiley & Sons, Inc., 1999.
7.   Young KD, Lewis RJ. What is confidence? Part 1: The use and interpretation of confidence intervals. *Annals of Emergency Medicine.* 1997;30:307-310.

How to Perform a Randomized Controlled Trial

Kemal I. Deen & M. T. P. R. Perera

Introduction

A prospective randomized trial is an experiment that is designed to provide the most accurate evidence, without bias, of a previously untested new treatment. Evidence gathered from a randomized trial is considered level 1 evidence. The aim of experimental design in a randomized trial is to ensure that all factors in the treatment group and control group of the experiment are equal except for the end-points being evaluated in the trial. The results of such a trial should, therefore, leave little to chance occurrence, usually referred to as error.

In this chapter, we describe preparation for a randomized trial, conduct of the trial and the methods available for report of its result.

Preparation

At the outset it is essential to understand that the end result of your trial will depend on the state of preparation. Hence, time spent at this stage of the experiment is usually directly proportional to the validity of your data and conclusions. The design should aim to be simple. Always aim to compare like with like, i.e. "apples with apples". Anything less will reduce the power of your conclusions. Foremost in the preparation is determination of the number of subjects required to provide a valid result that may be deemed significant with a 95%

confidence interval. This would require computation of a power to the study. Usually, a power level of 80% is the minimum acceptable standard that would ensure likelihood of little or no chance occurrence and that the conclusion is valid. An increase in your power, therefore, increases the validity of your conclusions. Most of the time, a power calculation may be obtained from a standard statistical package, as described in the chapter on statistics (Chapter 5). Once the power of your study is known, you will have the number of subjects required for evaluation. This number is final and should not be reduced in any way as a means of concluding the study. A randomized controlled trial may only be terminated in rare situations where the new treatment is either exceedingly beneficial, that makes the treatment of the control group unethical or where the new treatment is resulting in undue risk to the treatment group that makes continuation of the experiment dangerous.

Selection of Subjects

To achieve uniformity of both groups in the study, it is essential to define criteria for selection. These criteria that would enable inclusion of subjects in the study should be carefully thought out at the outset. It would be futile at the end of your experiment to realize that you have compared "apples with oranges"! For example, in a study designed to evaluate the value of internal anal sphincter repair in women with faecal incontinence after obstetric trauma, all women recruited to the study should have had obstetric trauma preceding incontinence as the primary criterion. Those who may have had previous haemorrhoidal excision, manual dilatation of the anal canal, internal sphincterotomy for fissure or any other cause for incontinence are unlikely to be suitable candidates. Because obstetric anal sphincter injury is unlikely to be associated with an isolated internal anal sphincter injury alone, we may encounter a number of recruitable women with concomitant external and internal anal sphincter injury. A study which sets out to include only those with isolated internal sphincter injury will not generate sufficient numbers and is impractical. However, while inclusion of those with combined internal and external anal sphincter injury will ascertain a satisfactory power to the study, it is important to ensure that there are similar numbers of women with combined anal sphincter damage in both test and control groups. The process of stratification will ensure similarity of both groups. Thus far, the experimental design will include all women of childbearing age (therefore, age and gender matched in both arms of the study) with anal incontinence after obstetric trauma. Possible exclusion criteria would be anal sphincter trauma due to non-obstetric causes. Stratification of those included for study based on the presence of concomitant external anal sphincter injury would establish similar proportions of these women in both treatment and control arms.

End Points

The end points of the experiment must be thought out at the time of commencement. Usually, these consist of the main outcome (primary end-point) and secondary outcomes (secondary end-points). An agreed primary end-point might be the degree of symptomatic improvement of incontinence based on an incontinence score. Secondary end-points may be change in anal sphincter pressures before and after surgical repair, and in the quality of life of these women.

Method of Randomization

Historically, to ensure equal distribution randomization had been performed with the toss of a coin. This underscores the principle of randomization, where the chance of a woman being recruited to either the treatment group or control group becomes equal. Thus, randomization is the key step that ensures both groups of the experiment are comparable. In the pre-computer era, randomization was performed using random tables. Currently, randomization is performed using computer generated random numbers. Computer generated random numbers also enable "fine tuning" of the process of randomization by allowing for random allocation in small groups, and by stratification. Randomization in small groups or blocks ensures better control of the process of equal distribution which may also facilitate cessation of a randomized trial, if so desired. For instance, if the total number of women needed to determine the efficacy of internal anal sphincter repair after obstetric trauma is 120, it would be better to randomize recruits in twelve blocks of ten each rather than incorporating a randomization protocol for the entire lot. Also, small groups are more manageable during the conduct of the study.

To better understand stratification of subjects, it would be convenient to consider the analogy of "apple with apple". Although random allocation would ensure inclusion of an "apple" in both treatment and control groups, it does not necessitate inclusion of only "red apples" in both groups, thus leaving room for bias. If the group available for selection does include the occasional "green apple", then stratification will ensure that the green apples, albeit a few, are distributed in similar numbers amongst the two groups available for study. Similarly, in the instance of women with obstetric anal incontinence, stratified randomization might enable equal distribution of those with combined external and internal anal sphincter injury in the study originally designed to evaluate the impact of surgical repair of the internal anal sphincter after obstetric trauma. Commercially available computer programs designed for random allocation also possess the stratification function.

Protocol, Pro-forma and Consent

Once the design of the study, method of recruitment, selection of subjects including end-points have been determined, which should also include total number required for accrual and the power of the study, it now becomes essential to incorporate all data, inclusion and exclusion criteria, in a pro-forma for each of the subjects. A well constructed pro-forma should also include a brief description of the purpose of the study and a flow chart of events which should help orientate all members of the research team. Finally, before commencement of the study, it is legally binding to have the study approved by a research ethics committee or institutional review board. The consent for study, which must be obtained in the case of all experimental subjects, must aim to have the background, purpose of study and likely advantages and disadvantages of being recruited to either of the treatment groups. The consent must be written in simple and clear language. It is a good practice to have the consent form read by several laypersons before submission of the study for ethical committee approval. Their advice is invaluable and any suggestions for alteration of consent must be given serious consideration. In the case of human subjects, it is essential for a consent form to state that the individual being evaluated would be free to choose to drop out of the study without being subject to treatment bias in the future. Purposeful groundwork in preparation of the consent will establish the foundation for sufficient number of accruals and a successful study.

Conduct of the Experiment

After successful vetting of the protocol by the ethical committee, it is now time to commence the much awaited experimental trial. Generally, it is helpful to appoint a trial coordinator, who may require a fee for services. A trial coordinator's job is to ensure smooth conduct of the trial. The coordinator, who should, ideally, not be a part of the active research team, helps relieve busy surgical trainees from the mundane chores of a trial such as speaking with members of multi-centre teams and being available to assist with random allocation of study subjects. This also helps in eliminating bias in random allocation to treatment or control arms of the study. Throughout the study, it is essential to look for bias and eliminate it. For instance, random allocation numbers must be enclosed within sealed envelopes where the option of allocation to treatment or control group must be decided at the time of executing the treatment. If the trial is aimed at comparing direct apposition sphincteroplasty with overlapping sphincteroplasty, the sealed envelope determining the type of operation should be disclosed only after skin incision, just before undertaking sphincter repair.

Documentation of Results

Again, elimination of bias should be the goal. The end-points of the trial should be assessed by an independent person who is not part of the operating team. Such a person might be a suitably qualified nurse or doctor who is blinded to the type of treatment administered to each individual in the study. Thus, names of individuals are best replaced by codes and type of treatment not included in the data sheet for documenting results of the study. The key to the codes must be secure in the hands of the coordinator. Inclusion of a suitably qualified independent observer of the trial is known to improve the quality of the results. Such persons often facilitate ethical conduct of trials.

Evaluation

All data obtained during the trial must be entered into data sheets in real time. Such entries are preferred in ink, such that an entry, once made, must not and cannot be altered in any way. It is helpful to evaluate early results of the trial as the experiment progresses after specific numbers have been recruited. After being included in a specific arm of a randomized study, the subject, for all intents and purposes must stay randomized to that specific arm and, more importantly, to the specific random number, even if the subject will not be included for future evaluation for any reason. For instance, If Ms. X was recruited as the 25th selection to treatment A, and wishes not to continue in the study, Ms. X must stay randomized to random number 25. The next subject recruited will be random number 26, not 25. Thus, although during recruitment, equal numbers of subjects may have been included in both arms of the experiment, comparison of trial results may not necessarily have equal numbers of subjects being evaluated because of attrition.

Termination of the Trial

A randomized controlled trial will usually yield accurate results only if completed as planned. In unusual circumstances, researchers may be compelled to terminate a trial prematurely. These situations are: if the new treatment under evaluation has proven to be harmful to subjects in the study that makes continuation of the study unsafe, or if the new treatment bears a result that exceeds expectation, by far, and where, by consensus, it is felt that continuation of the trial may be disadvantageous to those in the control group of the study. Rarely, if accrual becomes difficult and is insufficient, researchers may be compelled to retract from achieving the primary end-point of the study but may report no difference in the study groups, which may, in some instances, be a valid conclusion.[1]

Report of the Trial Result

During evaluation and report of the trial, the statistical expert must assume charge. Once evaluation has been undertaken, it is now time to report the preliminary result of the trial. This is usually done by way of verbal communication at various scientific meetings. Critique of the data during scientific meetings by experts in the field of study often prove to be important means of polishing the data and, eventually, in achieving a well written scientific manuscript for publication. Inclusion of a flow chart to demonstrate the progress of the trial complements the narrative when reporting and is known to improve the clarity of the study.[2]

Conclusion

The randomized trial has established itself as the standard against which all other experiments must be measured. The power remains the most vital factor. Selection of experimental subjects must attempt to eliminate bias at every stage of the study and both the researcher and study subjects should be blinded to the type of treatment administered, whenever possible. Every effort should be made to see a randomized trial to its end. Such trials are time consuming. The eagerness to publish early results by conclusion of a study must be resisted. The result of a randomized trial will provide level 1 evidence for practice.

References

1.   Nelson H et al. A comparison of laparoscopically assisted and open colectomy for colon cancer. *New Engl J of Med.* 2004; 350: 2050 - 2059.
2.   Sauer R, Becker H, Hohenberger W et al. Pre-operative versus post-operative chemoradiotherapy for rectal cancer. *New Engl J of Med.* 2004; 351: 1731 - 1740.

7

Cohort and Case Control Studies

S. R. E. Wijesuriya & M. H. J. Ariyaratne

Introduction

Epidemiological studies are conducted with the aim of investigating the relationship between exposure to a risk factor and development of a disease or a condition. Two basic designs can be used: case control studies and cohort studies. The fundamental difference between these two designs is that a case control study is initiated with cases or disease to identify causes or etiology if there are any, while cohort studies begin with a defined normal population which is followed up until the disease develops. The main drawback of observational studies is that they are non- randomized. However, these studies are useful when randomized control trials are either not feasible or unethical.

In conducting an observational study, a hypothesis should be formulated first, followed by data collection and finally by testing the hypothesis using a statistical method. (e.g. chi-square test)

Case Control Studies

In case control studies, comparisons are made between individuals who have a disease or a condition with those who do not have this particular condition. Hence, the starting point of a case control study is a particular disease or condition (cases). Once the cases are selected, a sample of individuals should be selected who do not have this particular disease or condition (controls). Subsequently, details regarding exposure are obtained by interview, or other sources.

Similarly, controls are also interviewed to assess the exposure and, if possible, to quantify it.

To avoid bias and problems during interpretation of data, cases that are selected should be newly diagnosed and both the cases and the etiological factors should be accurately defined. Selection of controls is one of the most difficult parts of a case control study. A random sample from the general population is selected, and this should be representative of the general population without the disease.

Exposure factors may be physiological characteristics of an individual such as sex or body mass index; personnel habits such as diet or tobacco smoking; occupational or environmental factors.

Case control studies can be either hospital based or population based.

Measure of association between disease and exposure

In case control studies, the association between etiological agents and the disease is given by the term odds ratio. Unlike in a prospective study, in case control studies, the absolute risk cannot be calculated. If it is assumed that the cases and the controls are random samples from their respective populations and that newly diagnosed cases are included in the study, approximate estimate of relative risk can be given and this is known as the odds ratio.

$$\text{Odds ratio} = \frac{\text{Odds of exposure in diseased subjects}}{\text{Odds of exposure in healthy controls}}$$

Exposure	With disease (cases)	Without disease (controls)	
Yes	a	b	a + b
No	c	d	c + d
	a + c	b + d	

Odds of exposure in diseased subjects = a/ c
Odds of exposure in healthy controls = b/d

$$\text{Odds ratio} = \frac{a/c}{b/d}$$

An example of a case control study is a northern Italian study to assess the role of alcohol consumption as an etiological factor of colorectal cancer.[1] This study had been conducted from 1985 to 1990 in the northern part of Italy, on 889 cases of colon cancer, 581 cases of rectal cancer, and 2,475 controls admitted to hospital for acute, non-neoplastic, non-digestive disorders. After obtaining necessary information no significant associations between alcohol intake and the risk of cancer of the colon or rectum were found.

In most case control studies there could be other factors which may directly or indirectly have an impact on occurrence of the disease under study. These factors are known as confounding factors. In the above example, in addition to alcohol there could be other confounding factors such as age, sex, body mass index, and other dietary habits which may have an impact on the final outcome. In such situations, either controls have to be matched for confounding factors (matched case control studies), or a computer-aided method can be employed to analyze data (SAS program).

Advantages of case control study

1   May be conducted over relatively short periods of time.
2   A good study design for a rare disease or a disease with a long latency between exposure and disease.
3   Multiple etiological factors can be assessed.
4   It is relatively more cost effective.

Disadvantages of case control study

1   Information regarding exposure to etiological agent is solely based on the memory of the individual; therefore, conclusions may be unreliable. (*Comparability*: inaccuracy in recall can affect the two groups to different degrees; *Validity*: recall may not reflect the true level of exposure.)
2   Does not provide incidence rate of the disease.
3   One disease can be studied at a time.
4   Control group may not always be appropriate.

Cohort Studies

In contrast to case control studies, cohort studies are commenced by employing healthy subjects. They are divided into two groups, who are exposed and not exposed respectively to a particular etiological agent or factor. Both groups are followed up prospectively until they develop the predetermined disease.

Outcome of a cohort study

There are two possible measurements upon conclusion of a cohort study.

1 Incidence rate, which can be defined as the proportion of individuals who develop the disease within the specified period of time.

2 Relative risk, which is the ratio of the incidence of disease in the exposed group and the non-exposed group.

Exposure	With disease (cases)	Without disease (controls)	
Yes	a	b	a + b
No	c	d	c + d
	a + c	b + d	

$$\text{Relative risk} = \frac{a / (a + b)}{c / (c + d)}$$

An example of a prospective cohort study is a study conducted in China to assess the association between alcohol consumption and the risk of colorectal cancer (CRC) in Chinese population. Chen et al.[2] conducted a population-based prospective cohort study during the period 1989-2001. Drinking habits of individuals were investigated with demographic information. The cohort was followed up and censored at the date of diagnosis of colorectal cancer, at death from any causes, or at the termination of the study, whichever came first. Of the individuals who were recruited to the study 64,100 individuals had finished the followup. Two hundred and forty two colorectal cancer patients were diagnosed during the study period. They were observed to have exhibited no significant association between alcohol consumption and the risk of colorectal cancer.

Advantages of a cohort study

1 Both the incidence and the relative risk can be calculated.
2 Information regarding exposure is obtained prospectively; therefore, it is more reliable than that in case control studies.

3 Multiple outcomes in relation to a single exposure can be assessed.

4 It is possible to study exposures which are rare.

Disadvantages of a cohort study

1 It is not a good method when a relatively rare disease is being studied.

2 Follow-up of a large number of patients may be difficult.

3 It is expensive and time consuming.

4 It may not be appropriate when there is a longer latent interval between exposure and the disease.

Bias Associated with Observational Studies

Bias is generally defined as a systematic error that results in an incorrect estimation of association between exposure and the disease.

One of the main biases associated with observational studies is the selection bias. There are several ways that a selection bias could occur. This may result due to error in sampling; as a result of refusal in participation, non-response or loss for follow-up in cohort studies. In addition, there could be associated bias during retrieval of information either during interview or recall.

Bias can be minimized by careful pre-planning which includes proper definitions of cases and controls, selection of both the cases and controls from the same population, standardizing the instruments of measurement and training of interviewers. Enrolling multiple controls and obtaining information using several sources (rather than recall only) may also help in minimizing bias in observational studies.

References

1. Barra S, Negri E, Franceschi S, Guarneri S, La Vecchia C. Alcohol and colorectal cancer: a case-control study from northern Italy. *Cancer Causes Control*. 1992 Mar;3(2):153-9.

2. Chen K, Jiang Q, Ma X, Li Q, Yao K, Yu W, Zheng S. Alcohol drinking and colorectal cancer: a population-based prospective cohort study in China. *Eur J Epidemiol*. 2005;20(2):149-54.

Meta-analysis Simplified

A. R. Wickremasinghe & A. Pathmeswaran

Introduction

This chapter provides a brief overview of meta-analysis and provides templates to conduct simple meta-analyses for selected effect measures. Statistical theory and derivation are not covered, but sources of such information have been included for the interested reader.

What is Meta-analysis?

A meta-analysis is a statistical analysis of a collection of studies. Huque defines meta-analysis as "A statistical analysis that combines or integrates the results of several independent clinical trials considered by the analyst to be 'combinable'.[1] Meta-analyses are done in the hope of identifying consistent patterns and sources of disagreement among results of studies.[2]

Meta-analysis is essentially synthesis of available data in the literature about a topic. Ideally, synthesis of randomized trials is carried out to arrive at a single summary estimate. Although Karl Pearson[3] is credited to be the first to pool results from separate studies in 1904, the term meta-analysis was coined in 1976 by the psychologist Glass.[4] Even though meta-analysis is used widely, it is still a controversial topic. The point of controversy is whether the primary objective of a meta-analysis should be estimation of an overall summary or average effect across studies (also referred to as a synthetic goal), or identification and estimation of differences among study-specific effects (an analytic goal). For clinicians, the former, i.e. the synthetic goal is the primary objective to decide on what treatment is best for the patient.

The Need for Meta-analysis

A single study often cannot detect or exclude with certainty a modest, albeit clinically relevant, difference in the effects of two treatments. A trial may show no significant treatment effect when such an effect truly exists, i.e. may produce a false negative result. This is also referred to as a type II error. Large sample sizes are generally required for minimizing type II errors which often cannot be achieved in a single study for cost considerations and even logistic reasons.

The meta-analytic approach is an attractive alternative to such a large, expensive, and logistically problematic study. Data of trials evaluating the same or a similar drug in several smaller, but comparable, studies are considered so that the necessary number of subjects is available to detect or exclude relatively small effects with confidence.

Meta-analysis enables the generalization of results to some degree. The findings of a particular study may be valid only for a population of patients with the same characteristics as those investigated in the trial. If many trials exist in different groups of patients, and similar results are obtained in the different trials, then it can be concluded that the effects of the intervention are similar across many populations and that they have some generality. In contrast, meta-analyses can also be used to answer some questions better than individual trials; for example, whether an overall study result varies among subgroups such as men and women, older and younger patients, or subjects with different degrees of severity of the disease.

Meta-analysis provides an opportunity for testing new hypothesis not posed in individual studies. It also provides a "more transparent appraisal" in that a quantitative component, that can be reproduced, is used.

Traditional Narrative Reviews

Traditional narrative reviews are no longer the simplest or the most reliable method of summarizing data. Besides, these are subjective and, therefore, prone to bias and error.[5] Reviewers can disagree on many issues including the types of studies to be included and how to balance the quantitative evidence they provide. Selective inclusion of studies that support the author's view is common. Likewise, the results of clinical trials in line with prevailing opinion are more likely to be cited than unsupportive studies.[6, 7]

Deciding on a set of studies to be reviewed is an important step in a meta-analysis. Once the set of studies has been decided upon, traditional reviews usually count the number of studies supporting various aspects of an issue and conclude with the view receiving the most votes. Such a procedure ignores sample size, effect size, and research design. Very often, this type of review gives opposite conclusions. Meta-analytic techniques currently available allow a more objective appraisal by integrating actual evidence.

Initial Steps in Performing a Meta-analysis

The most important initial step in conducting a meta-analysis consists of developing a research question. Once the research question is decided upon, the next task is to identify studies relating to that topic. This may be done by searching computerized databases such as Medline. After identifying all studies, define the ones you want to use in the meta-analysis. The decision whether to use the results of a particular study will depend on whether those studies do or do not match your requirements. The steps in a meta-analysis are given as a flow chart in Fig. 8.1.

Publication bias refers to the greater likelihood of research with statistically significant results being reported in comparison to those with null or non-significant results. In retrieving published data, this form of bias may be particularly important and the problem should be acknowledged in the study report.

It is essential that up-to-date material be reviewed to make optimal use of meta-analysis. The cut-off dates should be mentioned in the analysis so that the precise time period of the review is known to the reader. Likewise, if you are including only English language articles in the study, the rationale for doing so should also be stated.

If there are multiple reports published from the same study on the same topic, be sure to include only one study so that information from the same study population will not be duplicated in the analysis. It is better to exclude studies with small sample sizes to avoid overemphasizing small studies. Similarly, make an early decision about the period of follow-up of studies.

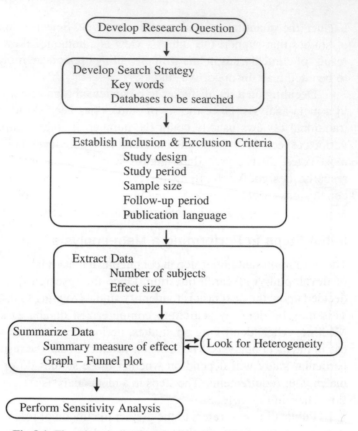

Fig 8.1. Flowchart indicating the steps in a meta-analysis

An early decision has to be made on whether you intend to include studies with similar exposures or outcomes in your analysis. This decision should be based on your experience and understanding of the research question. If you are too restrictive, you gain face validity, though you may end up omitting important studies.

The next step is to create structured formats to key in information taken from the selected studies. The structured formats will depend on the effect measure to be calculated. Structured formats for different effect measures are given in the examples (Tables 8.1-8.4).

If both randomized and non-randomized studies are reviewed in the same meta-analysis, the effect sizes should be reported separately for the randomized and non-randomized studies as the

Table 8.1. Meta-analysis calculations when effect measure is the relative risk

Study	Relative Risk Estimate	Upper Limit (RRu)	Lower Limit (RRl)	RRu/RRl	LnRR	VarRR [(LN(RR)/1.96)**2]	Weight (1/VarRR)	Weight* LnRR
1	1.12	1.60	0.75	2.13	0.76	0.15	6.69	5.07
2	1.69	2.00	1.32	1.52	0.42	0.04	22.25	9.25
3	0.72	2.50	0.06	41.67	3.73	3.62	0.28	1.03
4	0.91	1.32	0.65	2.03	0.71	0.13	7.65	5.42
5	1.01	1.45	0.65	2.23	0.80	0.17	5.97	4.79
Total							42.84	25.56

LnRR = ln (RRu/RRl)

LnRRS = (Total weight*LnRR)/(Total weight) = 25.56/42.84 = 0.60

VarRRs = 1/(Total weight) = 1/42.84 = 0.02

SqrtvarRRs = (VarRR)**(1/2) = 0.02**(1/2) = 0.15

LnRRS upper = (LnRRS + (1.96*SqrtvarRRs)) = (0.60 + (1.96*0.15)) = 0.90

LnRRS lower = (LnRRS - (1.96*SqrtvarRRs)) = (0.60 - (1.96*0.15)) = 0.30

Summary Relative Risk = exp (LnRRS) = exp (0.60) = 1.82

95% confidence interval (upper) = exp (LnRRS upper) = exp (0.90) = 2.45

95% confidence interval (lower) = exp (LnRRS lower) = exp (0.30) = 1.32

Table 8.2. Meta-analysis calculations for randomized control trials using Peto's method

Study	Events Treatment group (A)	Events Control group (B)	Non-events Treatment group (C)	Non-events Control group (D)	Total(T)	E {[(A+C)*(A+B)]/T}	Difference (A-E)	Var {[E*(B+D)*(A+C)]/[(T)*(T-1)]}
1	150	265	1350	1235	3000	207.50	-57.50	89.43
2	75	180	225	120	600	127.50	-52.50	36.72
3	30	40	120	110	300	35.00	-5.00	13.46
4	250	200	500	450	1400	241.07	8.93	76.00
5	92	102	670	700	700	94.52	-2.52	42.48
Sum							-108.59	258.09

T = Total = A + B + C + D

Peto's Odds Ratio (POR) = exp ((sum difference)/(sum var)) = -108.59 / 258.09 = 0.66

95% confidence interval upper = POR + ((1.96)/((258.09)**(1/2))) = 0.66 + (1.96/sqrt (258.09)) = 0.78

95% confidence interval lower = POR - ((1.96)/((258.09)**(1/2))) = 0.66 - (1.96/sqrt (258.09)) = 0.53

Table 8.3. Meta-analysis calculations for randomized control trials using the Mantel Haenszel method

Study	D-E	D-NE	ND-E	ND-NE	Total	Var	Weights	OR	P	F	R	R²	S²	G	H
1	190	100	345	257	892	0.03	38.68	1.42	54.74	27.43	54.74	2996.70	1495.92	46.69	19.30
2	100	50	100	150	400	0.08	12.50	3.00	37.50	23.44	37.50	1406.25	156.25	21.88	4.69
3	40	60	90	120	310	0.06	17.42	0.89	15.48	7.99	15.48	239.75	303.43	16.48	8.43
4	80	60	175	250	565	0.05	18.58	1.90	35.40	20.68	35.40	1253.03	345.37	25.58	7.73
5	25	10	50	40	125	0.25	4.00	2.00	8.00	4.16	8.00	64.00	16.00	5.92	1.92
Sum							91.18		151.12	83.70	151.12	5959.74	2316.97	116.55	42.06

D-E = Diseased among exposed
D-NE = Diseased among non-exposed
ND-E = Non-diseased among exposed
ND-NE = Non-diseased among non-exposed
Total = (D-E) + (D-NE) + (ND-E) + (ND-NE)
Var = Total/((D-NE)*(ND-E))
Weights = (1/Var)
OR = Odds Ratio = ((D-E)*(ND-NE))/((D-NE)*(ND-E))
P = Product = (Weights*OR)
F = ((D-E)*(ND-NE)) * (((D-E)+(ND-NE))/(Total*Total))
R = ((D-E)*(ND-NE))/Total
R² = R*R
S² = (1/var)*(1/var)

G $= ((((D-E)*(ND-NE)) * ((D-NE)+(ND-E))) + (((D-NE)*(ND-E)) * ((D-E)+(ND-NE)))) / (Total*Total)$

H $= (((D-NE)*(ND-E)) * ((D-NE)+(ND-E))) / (Total*Total)$

Varmh $= (((\text{sum } F)/(2*(\text{sum } R^2)) + ((\text{sum } G)/(2*(\text{sum } R)*(\text{sum weights}))) + ((\text{sum } H)/(2*(\text{sum } S^2)))$
$((83.70/(2*5959.74)) + (116.55/(2*151.12*91.18)) + (42.06/(2*2316.97))) = 0.02$

Summary Odds Ratio (SOR) $= (\text{sum } P)/(\text{sum weights}) = 151.12 / 91.18 = 1.66$
95% confidence interval upper $= \exp(\ln(SOR) + (1.96*(\sqrt{varmh}))) = \exp(\ln(1.66) + (1.96*(\sqrt{0.02}))) = 2.19$
95% confidence interval lower $= \exp(\ln(SOR) - (1.96*(\sqrt{varmh}))) = \exp(\ln(1.66) - (1.96*(\sqrt{0.02}))) = 1.25$

Table 8.4. Meta-analysis calculations when effect measure is the cumulative incidence or the rate difference

Study	E-T	E-C	NE-T	NE-C	TT	TC	TE	TNE	T	IT	IC	RD	varRD	Weight	P
1	150	250	1350	1250	1500	1500	400	2600	3000	10.00	16.67	6.67	0.00015	6490.38	43269.23
2	50	100	150	100	200	200	150	250	400	25.00	50.00	25.00	0.00234	426.67	10666.67
3	40	70	60	30	100	100	110	90	200	40.00	70.00	30.00	0.00495	202.02	6060.61
4	125	180	500	550	625	730	305	1050	1355	20.00	24.66	4.67	0.00052	1930.43	8991.02
5	80	130	450	500	530	630	210	950	1160	15.09	20.63	5.54	0.00052	1941.47	10756.89
Sum														10990.97	79744.42

E-T = Events in treatment group
E-C = Events in control group
NE-T = Non-events in treatment group

NE-C	= Non-events in control group	
TT	= Total in treatment group = ((E-T) + (NE-T))	
TC	= Total in control group = ((E-C) + (NE-C))	
TE	= Total events = ((E-T) + (E-C))	
TNE	= Total non-events = ((NE-T) + (NE-C))	
T	= Grand Total = TE + TNE = ((E-T) + (E-C) + (NE-T) + (NE-C))	
IT	= Incidence in treatment group = (((E-T)/(TT))*100)	
IC	= Incidence in control group = (((E-C)/(TC))*100)	
RD	= Rate difference = IC – IT	
VarRD	= Variance of RD = ((TE*TNE)/(TT*TC*T))	
Weight	= 1/varRD	
P	= Product = (RD*weight)	
Varsum		= 1/(sum weights) = 1/10990.97 = 0.000091
Summed std.dev. (SSD)		= (SQRT(varsum)*100) = (SQRT(0.000091)*100) = 0.95
Summary rate difference (SRD)		= (sum P) / (sum weights) = 79744.42 / 10990.97 = 7.26
95% confidence interval upper		= ((SRD) + (1.96*(SSD))) = 7.26 + (1.96*0.95) = 9.13
95% confidence interval lower		= ((SRD) - (1.96*(SSD))) = 7.26 - (1.96*0.95) = 5.39

effect of a new treatment is likely to be larger in non-randomized studies.

Statistical Methods

Statistical analyses are performed to determine a summary effect estimate (a rate difference, an odds' ratio, relative risk or a rate ratio) and its confidence limits. The selection of an effects model is important. Usually, the choice is between a fixed effects model, indicating that the conclusions derived in the meta-analysis are valid for the studies included in the analysis, and a random effects model, assuming that the studies included in the meta-analysis belong to a random sample of a universe of such studies. When the studies are found to be homogeneous, random and fixed effects models are indistinguishable. A random effects model is computationally more intense than a fixed effects model. In this chapter, examples having simulated data of meta-analyses calculations for different effect measures are presented in templates derived from Basu[8] in Tables 8.1-8.4. Required information for the Tables is given in bold.

The determination of the summary effect measure is based on weighting the effect measures of individual studies based on sample sizes. The templates given in Tables 8.1-8.4 can be obtained from the web[8] or programmed in a Microsoft EXCEL worksheet.

Most studies are presented with many effect estimates and sub-analyses, and the choice of the effect estimate to be used may be difficult. In randomized control trials (RCTs), the estimate derived by intention to treat analysis should be taken. In non-randomized study designs, take estimates that are adjusted for age and established confounders.

Example 1 (Table 8.1)

In this example, the relative risk is the estimate of effect. This template can be used for prognostic studies. The effect estimate and the 95% confidence limits of individual studies have to be provided. The remaining intermediate variables can be calculated.

Examples 2 and 3 (Tables 8.2 and 8.3)

Examples 2 and 3 can be used interchangeably for randomized control trials. Peto's method (Table 8.2) is computationally simpler. The Mantel Haenszel method is a widely used method of stratified data analysis. Both methods cannot control for the effects of confounders.

For both methods, the 2x2 matrix for individual studies is required. The remaining intermediate variables can be calculated.

Example 4 (Table 8.4)

In this example, the cumulative incidence or the rate difference is the measure of effect. The 2 x 2 matrix for individual studies is required.

Graphical Methods

The funnel plot is a very useful graph in meta-analysis. It is a plot showing the effect size on the X-axis and the sample size on the Y-axis.[9] With smaller sample sizes, occurrence of wide differences in the effect size is possible and with increasing sample sizes the differences in the effect size decrease. This phenomenon gives an inverted funnel shape to the plot (Fig. 8.2). The plot can be used to graphically summarize the results of the studies included in the meta-analysis. In addition, it can be useful in demonstrating whether or not all relevant trials have been included in the meta-analysis.

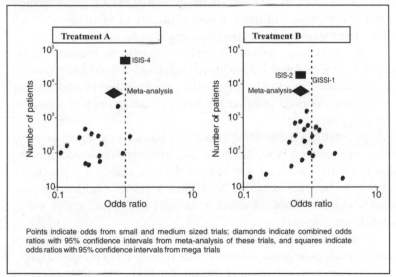

Points indicate odds from small and medium sized trials; diamonds indicate combined odds ratios with 95% confidence intervals from meta-analysis of these trials, and squares indicate odds ratios with 95% confidence intervals from mega trials

Fig. 8.2. Graphical methods of summarizing data: the funnel plot

Heterogeneity

Heterogeneity in meta-analysis refers to the variability of studies that are used for the analysis. Studies may differ in the patient groups studied, the intervention applied, the primary outcome examined and the settings in which the studies were carried out. The mixing of diverse studies casts doubts on the meaning of aggregate measures.

Graphical presentation of analyses of studies grouped by important variables (patient, intervention and setting characteristics) may give an idea of heterogeneity of studies. The Q-statistics, distributed as a chi square distribution with N-1 degrees of freedom (where N is the number of studies considered) can also be used to assess whether studies are homogenous (For more details refer to Petiti[10]). However, most statistical tests used to test for homogeneity of studies lack sufficient power to detect anything but substantial differences.[11] Simple 'eyeballing' of diversity of studies, common sense and clinical experience may be better guides.

Sensitivity Analysis

A sensitivity analysis should be conducted to test that the model you propose is a good model. The sensitivity analysis shows that results from a meta-analysis are robust to the choice of the statistical method and to the exclusion of trials of poorer quality or of studies stopped early. The extent of publication bias can also be assessed.[11]

In conducting a sensitivity analysis, firstly, the overall effect is calculated by different statistical methods (both a fixed and a random effects model). Virtually identical overall estimates and similar confidence intervals indicate relatively small amount of variation between trials.

Secondly, a methodological quality has to be assessed in terms of how patients are allocated to active treatment or control groups, how outcome is assessed, and how the data are analyzed.[12] The points scheme to be allotted has to be defined a priori. Exclusion of low quality studies should not affect drastically the overall effect and its confidence intervals.

Thirdly, stratification of the analysis by study size can identify publication bias as smaller effects can be significant in published larger studies. However, exclusion of the smaller studies has little effect on the overall estimate.

Studies stopped earlier than anticipated are likely to bias the results of the meta-analysis away from the null value. Exclusion of such studies should not drastically affect the overall estimate and its confidence limits if the model proposed is appropriate.

References

1. Huque MF. Experiences with meta-analysis in NDA submissions. *Proceedings of the Biopharmaceutical Section of the American Statistical Association.* 1988; 2: 28-33.
2. Rothman KJ, Greenland S. eds. *Modern Epidemiology.* 2nd Edition. Philadelphia: Lippincott Williams & Wilkins, 1998; 643-673.
3. Pearson K. Report on certain enteric fever inoculation statistics. *BMJ.* 1904; 3: 1243-6.
4. Glass G. Primary, secondary and meta-analysis of research. *Educ Res.* 1976; 5: 3-8.
5. Teagarden J R. Meta-analysis: whither narrative review? *Pharmacotherapy.* 1989; 9: 274-84.
6. Ravnskov U. Cholesterol lowering trials in coronary heart disease: frequency of citation and outcome. *BMJ.* 1992;305:15-9.
7. Götzsche P C. Reference bias in reports of drug trials. *BMJ.* 1987; 295: 654-6.
8. Basu A. How to conduct a meta-analysis. http://www.pitt.edu/AFShome/s/u/super1/public/html/lecture/lec1171/
9. Davies HTO, Crombie IK. What is Meta-analysis? Aventis House, Kent. Vol 1: Number 8.
10. Petiti DB. *Meta-analysis, Decision Analysis and Cost Effectiveness Analysis in Medicine.* New York: Oxford University Press, 1994.
11. Egger M, Smith GD, Phillips AN. Meta-analysis: principles and procedures. *BMJ.* 1997; 315: 1533-1537
12. Prendiville W, Elbourne D, Chalmers I. The effects of routine oxytocic administration in the management of the third stage of labour: an overview of the evidence from controlled trials. *Br J Obstet Gynaecol.* 1988; 95: 3-16..

How to Write an Abstract
Jason T. Lee & Ravin R. Kumar

Introduction

Writing the abstract is an integral part of surgical research and it requires precision and care. All phases of a research project are connected with writing of a clear abstract—submission of proposals for funding, presentation at a meeting, and final publication. The tone of the research project presentation is set with the abstract and a well-written abstract allows the researcher to efficiently present new knowledge and insights to colleagues. A concise, structured abstract is necessary for reviewers to evaluate the quality and merit of the project during presentations at surgical meetings and for publication in a journal. Learning to write an effective abstract is an essential skill for the academic surgeon and forms the basis for a successful research career. In this chapter, we review the basics of constructing an abstract including a discussion of the structure, content, language, and the submission process.

Organizing the Abstract

The abstract for a surgical research project should contain a brief introduction to the question or problem being studied, a clear hypothesis, the methods utilized to collect data, a review of the pertinent results, and the implications of the findings. In the surgical literature, a brief guideline to preparation of an organized abstract was described in 1976, calling for a general form to include an introduction, the data, and a concluding statement.[1] The concept of the structured abstract was proposed in 1987 in an attempt to provide a more informative description of clinical trials.[2] This model has been adapted in most medical journals and is formatted to include specific sections and brief statements of defined content. The headings of these sections that are included in most surgical journals are the Introduction/Background, Objectives, Methods, Results, and Conclusions.

Structured abstracts have numerous advantages over the traditional descriptive paragraph seen at the beginning of older medical literature. They are easier to read and search because the text is opened up and clearly subdivided into consistent parts.[3] Readers are more able to select valid and applicable articles while reading structured abstracts, and the precision of computerized MEDLINE searches is improved. Many journals also have subcategories listed in the abstract to further alert the reader to the type of research being written about. Examples include the study design (i.e. prospective trial, retrospective review), setting and study population (i.e. private practice, academic referral center, rural), and main outcome measures. With the acceptance in the majority of medical journals of the structured abstract for clinical trials, different subheadings and criteria have also been proposed for review articles, grant submissions and clinical practice guidelines.[4]

What to Write in the Abstract

After you have organized your thoughts in terms of the structure of the abstract, the next step is to decide what information to include in each section. Guidelines have been prepared for the content to be included in the structured abstract.[5] Begin the abstract with a concise statement of the purpose of the project or study, including the exact question to be addressed by the project. If you have a hypothesis, be sure that it is clearly stated. Remember that the reviewer may not be an expert in the field you are studying and reporting on, so a sentence to explain the significance and relevance of your work is helpful. Use the introduction and background portion to place your project in the context of the broad research question. The challenge is to convey the information in a few well-chosen sentences as to why your contribution is potentially important without spending too many words stating universally accepted facts.[6]

After introducing your topic, describe the design and methods utilized in your study. Again, the challenge lies in deciding how much information to provide to enable the reader/reviewer to judge the applicability of your methods and subsequent findings and conclusions. Describe very clearly the techniques, treatments, or interventions that were fundamental to obtaining your data. For clinical studies, the location and setting of the hospital, how patients were accrued, whether data were obtained prospectively or retrospectively, and randomization protocols are important in demonstrating the strength of your research design. Statistical methods utilized can also be mentioned in this section, which typically add validity to your work.

The results should be where the bulk of your word limit is used up. State in as much detail the outcome measures, numerical findings, and statistical significance with P-values. Accepted abstracts will typically be judged to have better content because of more accurate numerical and statistical data.[7] Describe data that directly support or invalidate the hypothesis posed in your introduction. Note whether there were any other interesting findings that are clinically relevant or that came up unexpectedly. And finally, if the data were not available when the abstract was due, do not write that "analysis is to be performed"; simply, do not submit the abstract.

In the last section of your abstract, draw conclusions from your data. Summarize the findings, explain what they possibly mean, and indicate why it is important for other surgeons to have this new knowledge. Note whether there are direct clinical applications of your findings. Be sure to recognize the limitations of your study and never make claims beyond what your data can support. If there is a "take-home message", then clearly state it in the final sentence.

Wording of the Abstract

The language of the abstract is as vital as its structure and content. Sufficient time and effort need to be devoted by the academic surgeon in honing his writing skills in order to create an informative, yet concise abstract that conveys to the readers, many of whom are busy clinicians, a brief overview of the research project. One major hurdle often encountered in writing the abstract is the space limitation; usually, the upper limit is 250 words. These space limitations were designed not only for the convenience of bringing out a single program book to be given to all attendees of a surgical meeting, but also for the convenience of the busy group of reviewers who are required to read through the large number of submissions in a short amount of time and select those worthy of presentation. Early drafts are often too long, and require multiple rewrites and advice from co-authors to create the most effective abstract.

Proper wording of the abstract aids in the clarity of presentation. Numerous guidelines on how to write clear abstracts and more readable medical text have been written.[3] Terminology used should be uniformly accepted and recognized by surgeons, and devoid of confusing abbreviations or eponyms. The use of the third person should be minimized as far as possible, and active rather than passive tense should be utilized. Follow the rules of economy of language and simplicity of statement, and do not embellish your sentences. For example, do not write "These findings allow us to conclude that ..." when one can more simply write "We conclude ..." or "In conclusion..." Write in simple declarative sentences and avoid redundancy. Use Standard English and precise technical terms while following conventional grammar and punctuation rules. All these steps help in improving the readability and clarity of the abstract without detracting from the significance of good surgical research.

As important as selection of your words carefully in the body of the abstract is the choice of a title. The title should be an attempt, in as few words as possible, to attract the attention of the reader without exaggerating the facts of the research. The title should also aid the program committee in placing the abstract in the appropriate part of the meeting, should it be accepted. Finally, the abstract title is utilized in most search engines of medical literature, and should have useful keywords so that literature searches will locate your abstract.

Sending in the Abstract

Timely submission of an abstract is the key to maximizing chances of its acceptance for a meeting. Late submissions are nearly always rejected, as are those that do not follow the guidelines.[8] Formatting rules are usually outlined in the notice calling for abstracts along with an abstract submission form. There is usually a range of acceptable topics, formatting and size requirements for the submission, a word limit, and most importantly, the deadline. Be sure that the abstract fits into the borders of the box that is usually provided and use the recommended font size and section headings. More recently, online abstract submission has become more popular and more convenient, offering automatic word counting and formatting according to the structure accepted by the organizers of the meeting. Remember that meeting organizers desire optimal abstracts to improve the overall quality of the scientific session and stimulate academic interest.

Conclusion

The basic purpose for gathering at annual meetings is sharing of new knowledge and insights with other surgeons. Writing an abstract, preparing the presentation, and submitting a paper are all essential tools in disseminating such knowledge. With the overwhelming amount of surgical research, technological advances, and multitude of surgical journals in print, it is often difficult to stay completely current. The abstract becomes a very influential stand-alone document in that it is more widely available on MEDLINE and is often the only part of an article that is read. A succinct abstract provides an efficient tool in summarizing new findings for our colleagues. In summary, being able to write an effective abstract is a crucial skill for the surgical researcher for obtaining funding, making presentations at national meetings, and publishing in peer-reviewed journals.

References

1. Warren R. The good abstract. *Arch Surg.* 1976;111:635-636.
2. Ad hoc working group for critical appraisal of the medical literature. A proposal for more informative abstracts of clinical articles. *Ann Intern Med.* 1987;106:598-604.
3. Hartley J. Clarifying the abstracts of systematic literature reviews. *Bull Med Library Assoc.* 2000;88:332-337.
4. Tenenbein M. The abstract and the academic clinician. *Pediatr Emerg Care.* 1995;11:40-42.
5. Haynes RB, Mulrow CD, Huth EJ, Altman DG, Gardner MJ. More informative abstracts revisited. *Ann Intern Med.* 1990;113:69-76.
6. Kraft AR, Collins JA, Carey LC, Skinner DB. Art and logic in scientific communication: abstracts, presentations and manuscripts. *J Surg Res.* 1979;26:591-604.
7. Panush RS, Delafuente JC, Connelly CS, Edwards NL, Greer JM, Longley S, et al. Profile of a meeting: how abstracts are written and reviewed. *J Rheumatol.* 1989;16:145-147.
8. McNamara, Grannell M, Watson RG, Bouchier-Hayes DJ. The research abstract: worth getting it right. *Ir J Med Sci.* 2001;170:38-40.

How to Make an Oral Presentation

F. R. Fernando

Introduction

Oral presentation is a very important method of communication. Successful people, either in business or in a profession, possess the ability to communicate well. They are able to transmit the exact message in a way that will be well received and understood. The persuasive power of an oral presentation must not be underestimated. It is a skill every doctor must posses.

Over one-half of an oral message is actually communicated visually. Hence, the slides and speech must be synchronized. It is imperative that the speaker establishes a 'rapport' with the audience at the start. Some speakers have the innate ability to do this while others need to develop the art.

Steps that ensure the success of a presentation are: *preparation* and *competent delivery*.

Preparation

There are several stages in preparation:
1. Formulating a clear plan and making the presentation easy to understand.
2. Careful preparation of presentations - slides/visual aids.
3. Rehearsal of the presentation.

Formulating a clear plan

The following thoughts may help in formulating a clear plan:

- What is the message you wish to deliver?
- Do you wish to inform, persuade or entertain!? – (Scientific presentation is about the first and the second.)
- How best can you organize your data to support your message?
- Are your conclusions valid?
- Do you want to "provoke" questions?

Work out in your mind what you want to say and the best method of saying it. Write down a plan and an outline of the speech. Read and reference the topic thoroughly. You should understand the presentation very well. If you do, the audience is likely to do so too. Try to cater to the simplest 'mind' in the audience. You can make a very detailed and high-sounding presentation, but if the audience fails to understand, it will be a completely worthless effort.

Preparation of your presentation

Following are some simple rules to follow:

- Slides must be prepared with a standard software package (e.g. PowerPoint). This will ensure trouble-free presentation.
- Keep the background uniform. This minimizes distraction.
- Use multimedia effects sparingly to limit distraction (remember it is a scientific presentation not a demonstration of multimedia techniques!)
- Use capitals sparingly. This maintains the correct emphasis.
- Use only one type of illustrations for a set of data, e.g. bar diagram, pie chart or graph. Do not use all three.
- Use of relevant references from the literature adds value to your presentation.
- All slides must have titles.
- Use a spell checker! Get someone else to check the slide show too.
- Try not to use too many colours which may distract the audience. Use standard fonts and a suitable font size (Arial 28 for slide text has been the best in my experience).
- Do not have more than 10 lines on a slide – no one can read a lot and listen at the same time!

Rehearsal of your presentation

However highly experienced you may be, it is necessary to rehearse the presentation several times. There are many ways of doing it. Some speakers practise in front of a mirror. Others simply present the talk to themselves and some others present the work to a person at home. Choose a method that best suits you. As you become more experienced, you will know how best to rehearse. It is essential to stay on-time; ensure your presentation ends within the time allocated; exceeding the time limit indicates poor preparation which risks irritating the audience and embarrassing the chairperson.

Competent Delivery

Try to create an impression from the time you walk up to the podium. Dress appropriately to suit the occasion. This varies from meeting to meeting and country to country. Do not be over-dressed or under-dressed. Walk unhurriedly and confidently. It helps the audience focus attention on you. Once on stage, look confident, stay close to the microphone and minimize movements. These ensure minimum distraction and the audience can hear you clearly.

From the moment you commence your speech, attempt to capture the attention of the audience. Some experienced and erudite speakers have the innate ability to do this. Eye contact with the audience is essential. The best way to establish eye contact is by looking directly at the audience or focusing at a point just above their heads.

The secret of successful presentation is simplicity. The value of a presentation is measured by what the audience grasps. So, keep it simple. Present information in sequence. Avoid flipping back and forth with the slides. The audience will find it disconcerting and difficult to follow you, thus losing interest.

Should you use humour? There are advantages and disadvantages. If humour comes naturally to you, use it. Otherwise, avoid it as it can distract and be off-putting. Tailor your humour to the audience, e.g. do not talk about cricket to an audience with many Japanese!

Any presentation has three basic components:
- **Introduction**
- **Body**
- **Conclusion**

Introduction

This is the critical part. 'Rapport' with the audience is established at this point. How should you do it? What should you say? Most speakers would introduce themselves and the institution and thank the organizers for the opportunity given to present the paper. Such mundane matters make life easy and are not controversial which helps break the ice. It is best to undertake introduction in this manner until sufficient experience has been gained. Synchronizing the introduction with a pretty picture of the hospital or the country you represent helps too. Now you are on your way!

Body

This is the main part of the presentation. Make use of the time allocated and present information in an unhurried, lucid and simple manner. Do not write everything on the slide. Rather, you should use the text on the slide as a cue.

The body of the scientific presentation should contain the following:

- Introduction - State the background information that prompted the study.
- Objective- Main purpose of the study.
- Study - What type of study it is, e.g. prospective randomized clinical trial.
- Patients and method - Study design, inclusion-exclusion criteria and statistical methods used.
- Findings - All the relevant information including statistical analysis. Don't be afraid to allude to weaknesses in your study (but don't over-emphasize these).

It is good practice to re-emphasize key findings during the presentation (for example, use of a different form of words) so that the audience remembers them.

Conclusion

- Conclusion should be precise, concise and well supported by data presented. Ideally, it should stimulate further study or prompt change in practice.
- You must try to convince the audience that your findings and conclusions have a scientific basis and are valid.

Answering Questions

There will usually be time for questions. Answering questions is an acquired talent! Never be afraid - it is simple for the uninitiated to ask a question! If you are well prepared you would have anticipated some of the questions and even prompted some. There are several techniques of responding to questions.

- Provide a direct answer - the best way!
- Use humour.
- Claim ignorance!
- Ask another question.
- Don't answer the question.

Whichever method you employ, try not to be arrogant or show annoyance. Most speakers become accomplished at answering questions after a few presentations under their belt.

Acknowledgements

Do not forget to thank the people who helped you with the study (including the patients) and those who helped in preparing the presentation. If the study was sponsored, the sponsors must be acknowledged. Most speakers tend to indicate conflicts of interest, particularly if the study had been sponsored by a pharmaceutical agency which has vested interests in the study. Finally, thank the audience for listening to the presentation. Good luck!

References

1. Katherine Jackson. Oral presentation. jacksok@hope.ac.uk, www.hope.ac.uk/gnu
2. Dennis S. Bernstein. Professor Bernstein's Top Ten Tips for Giving a Presentation. dsbacro@umich.edu
3. Marina Canapero. Guidelines for Scientific Presentations. www.frontier.iarc.uaf.edu:8080/~bhatt/atm693.f03.fall2002.

How to Write a Paper in the Medical Sciences

C. Goonaratna & H. J. de Silva

Introduction

One of the remarkable things we have learned by experience as editors
of a medical journal is that a carelessly disparaging comment about a
prospective author's article will often evoke a more irate riposte than
a similar remark, for example, about his or her clothes, car or home.
We think that the principal reason for such a vigorous reaction is not
so much authors' valuation of the crucial role of scientific research,
as the inherent value of a publication. The results of research that do
not achieve publication are of very limited import. Two famous
epigrams – "Work, finish, publish" (Faraday), and "The object of
science is publication" (Ziman) – epitomize the decisive role of
publication in the advancement of science as well as researchers'
careers.

Before the appearance of the *Philosophical Transactions of the
Royal Society* and *Journal de Scavans* in 1665, researchers had to
write a book or dispatch lengthy epistles to several fellow scientists
to spread the word about their research. Both forms of communication
were tedious, inefficient, and open to cribbing or wholesale plagiarism
of what we refer to nowadays as "intellectual property". Besides,
books and letters to fellow scientists gave researchers neither
opportunity to establish verifiable priority for their discoveries or
hypotheses, nor the benefit of reasonably brisk peer evaluation. The

emergence and proliferation of scientific journals have vastly changed things, we believe for the better. Publication of researchers' names and the dates on which articles were received establishes priority, openness to peer evaluation tends to confer authenticity, and subsequent citation ensures dissemination of their findings among a much wider readership. Scientific journals are now so numerous that almost all articles that scientists write get published somewhere.

What Do Editors Look For?

What do editors like to see in a scientific paper? They like newness (i.e. originality), trueness (i.e. sound methodology and valid interpretation of results), importance, and a flawless style. If your paper is on a fashionable topic and likely to generate some controversy, so much the better. Only a few papers that reach editors' desks will fulfil all these criteria to their satisfaction. If trueness of your paper is low, it is likely to be rejected. If the tests for newness, trueness and importance are passed, editors will usually not grudge spending time to improve the dreadful style of a paper. When the score for trueness is high, but the originality and importance of a paper are only so-so, an elegant style and neat presentation may tilt an editor's decision towards acceptance, because he is only human.

The overwhelming majority of authors who send their papers to journal editors think that the research they have done is of good quality, and that the paper ought to be accepted for publication. It is entirely natural that a large proportion of authors' self-assessments are overestimates. So, before starting to write your paper there are four questions that you should try to answer as objectively as you can.

1. Are the results of my research (or my case report, hypothesis, or review article) worth publishing?
2. Have I previously published these results in whole or in part elsewhere?
3. Who will be interested to read my paper?
4. What is the appropriate journal for my paper?

The second question is a test of your integrity. If your paper is wholly or in essence a duplicate publication, a good referee is likely to discover this because electronic bibliographic databases are now so freely accessible. If your paper gets published, some readers are sure to discover your ethical infraction and notify the journal editor, and other readers by a letter to the journal's correspondence section.

To answer the other three questions, it is useful to enlist the advice of a friendly but critical senior colleague. If your paper has a clear message that can be stated in one sentence, and it passes the trueness tests, it is likely to be accepted. Below are some examples of clear messages.

1. A new ACE-inhibitor B delays the progress of established diabetic nephropathy.
2. Statin C is better than statin D in lowering LDL-cholesterol.
3. Elective surgery for a prolapsed intervertebral disc is as good as emergency surgery even in the presence of urinary incontinence.

Most research will not yield such clear-cut and seminal messages. Editors will usually accept for publication papers that add even modestly to current knowledge, conflict with or confirm accepted ideas, or indicate improvements to clinical practice or health systems and so on, always provided that the paper has a message worth publishing, and has passed the trueness tests.

If you wish to report, for example, the results of 100 operations that you have performed for carcinoma of the pelvic colon, it is essential to ask yourself the question "What are the key points that I have to make?" If you are unable to state clearly at least two or three original key points, your paper is probably not worth publishing. Much retrospective "data dredging" masquerades as research. Reporting lots of data and your undoubtedly splendid experiences in the forlorn hope that some colleagues may be interested to read them is not a good enough reason for an editor to publish that paper. Data collection should be planned beforehand to answer a few relevant and clearly formulated questions if the exercise is to yield messages worth communicating in a scientific paper.

When the newness and trueness criteria are satisfied, and the paper has a clear message, editors may then apply the "So-what test" to decide on acceptance for publication. Your article is new, it is true and its message is clear: So what? Will your paper change clinical practice, health care systems, client perceptions, or scientific concepts? You are entitled to indicate your responses to the "So-what test" in the Discussion section (see below) of your paper. But please do not exaggerate the implications of your results; hyperbole sounds so hollow!

The answers to the third and fourth questions are closely related. If the message of your paper is only likely to interest cardiologists or paediatric neurologists, it will stand a much better chance of getting published if it is sent to an appropriate specialist journal. But such decisions may not always be straightforward. Consider a hypothetical paper on a small outbreak of a new fungal infection of the brain in a neonatal unit. Clearly, it may interest a much wider circle of readers than paediatric neurologists, for it may be of over-arching importance for epidemiologists, mycologists, clinical pharmacologists and immunologists, as well as for neurologists and paediatricians. If your paper is as important as that hypothetical one, it would be worth sending it to a prestigious general medical journal. But do remember that their rejection rates may be as high as 90%, mainly because they receive 2000 to 7000 papers each year, and can publish only a very few of them. Sometimes it is wise to sacrifice a little prestige for a much better chance of acceptance and quicker publication. After all, if your paper is an important one, and the less prestigious journal you have chosen is indexed, it is likely to be frequently cited.

Editors take a dim view of the so-called "salami publications"; that means a research paper sliced into several publications without good reason. The temptation to get several papers out of one research study derives from the need to fatten one's list of publications for promotions or landing more attractive positions. Decisions regarding multiple publications are difficult for editors. Going back to that hypothetical paper, it may have newly discovered culture methods appropriate for a journal of mycology or microbiology, unusual pharmacokinetics of an antifungal drug in neonates suitable for a journal of clinical pharmacology, previously unreported immunological deficiencies worth publishing in a journal of immunology, and so on. Taken all together, the paper will be far too long for one article. And there are legitimate reasons for sending the various parts of it to specialist journals, and only a summary clinical description to a prestigious general medical journal, citing your previous publications in specialist journals. But is there a valid case for slicing, for example, an essentially clinical study of Mycoplasma pneumoniae infection into three papers, one describing its pulmonary manifestations, another its neurological features, and a third its cardiovascular features?

The basic structure of a scientific paper is discussed beneath, followed by some notes on style.

Organizing the Content

Scientific journals require that the contents of a paper are organized in a uniform manner. Papers should include an Introduction (Why did you start?), Methods (What did you do?), Results (What did you find?) and Discussion (What does it mean?). In addition, most journals require an Abstract of the paper.

The title should be informative, specific, and retrievable. It should not be long or sensationalist. Short titles are clearer and catchy. Brevity could be achieved by eschewing adjectives and adverbs. Index words should be carefully selected, for they make it possible to retrieve the article from indices such as Index Medicus or Medline. It may be advisable to decide on a final title and index words last.

Introduction

Make the Introduction brief and to the point. It is not, as often thought, a detailed historical review of the topic. In the Introduction explain to the reader why you started the study and the hypothesis that was tested. The question(s) you have set out to answer (objectives) should be stated clearly and simply. To lead the reader to this point, a brief review of the relevant literature is necessary. In the literature review cite only papers that are essential to justify your objectives.

At the end of a good Introduction the reader ought to be clear regarding the question(s) you have set out to answer, and convinced that the question is an important one. It is usually an unsolved problem, or one where the evidence is equivocal.

Methods

The Methods section is an explanation of what exactly you did, e.g. definitions, ethical aspects, subjects and calculation of sample size, design and setting, duration, randomization, details of laboratory methods, statistics, etc. It should include descriptions of how subjects were recruited, criteria for exclusion, how randomization was done, materials and apparatus used, and where relevant, the doses of drugs. In short, the Methods section must be detailed enough to enable other suitably qualified readers to attempt to reproduce the work if they wish.

Results

The Results section should only include what was found that is relevant to the question(s) you set out to answer (objectives). Irrelevant data, however interesting they may seem, should not be included. The best (most reader-friendly) way to present data is usually an appropriate mix of text, tables and figures. Tables and figures should have legends that can stand alone. Prepare them according to the journal's instructions to authors.

Descriptive data or brief numerical results could be stated in the text. "There were 80 patients; their sex distribution is shown in the pie chart. Their ages ranged from 42 to 68 years," could be simply stated, "There were 80 patients (50 males) aged between 42 and 68 years." Numerical data requiring detailed description may be conveniently tabulated, e.g. there were 80 patients, 50 males and 30 females. Of the males, 10 smoked more than 40 cigarettes a day, 30 smoked 20-40 a day, 20 smoked 10-20 a day, 15 smoked 1-10 a day, and 5 did not smoke. Of the females, 5 smoked more than 40 cigarettes a day, 10 smoked 20-40 a day, 5 smoked 10-20 a day, 5 smoked 1-10 a day, and 5 did not smoke. This could be made easier to comprehend by tabulation (Table 11.1).

Table 11.1. Smoking among males and females

Number of cigarettes smoked per day	Males (n=50)	Females (n=30)
>40	10	5
20-40	30	10
10-20	20	5
1-10	15	5
0	5	5

Comparisons and relationships between sets of data are often best presented graphically (graphs or scatter plots). The data in the table below (Table 11.2) could also be presented graphically.

Table 11.2. Relationship between prostate cancer and age

Age group	Number with prostate cancer
(Years)	(n=345)
20-40	10
41-50	15
51-60	60
61-70	120
>71	140

Discussion

The discussion need not be an exhaustive review. You may briefly recapitulate the main findings, the methods used (especially if they were interesting or unusual), and any shortcomings in the methodology. The discussion is also the place to compare your results with those of other workers, whether they confirm or conflict with your results. If it is the latter case, possible reasons for the differences should be explained. The implications of your findings for future research, patient care, streamlining health systems, or modifying life styles and so on can be given as a succinct conclusion. Any recommendations that you make must be reasonable and justifiable by the results obtained.

Abstract

This is a summary of the chief points in the main body of the paper. It is the essence of your paper, and should be able to stand alone. Most journals place a 150 to 250 word limit on the abstract. Note that after the title, the abstract is the most read part of a paper; it may indeed be the only part. It is also the part that most editors read first. Hence, it is important to make it concise, readable and informative.

An abstract should contain all the essential information of a paper. That is to say, why the study was done, what was done, what was found, and what is concluded. There is no place in it for flowery language, details or discussion about anything. However, it should not be so absurdly short as to be unintelligible. The worst abstracts are those that end with the words "The results are discussed."

A good abstract is hard to write, so abstracts are often badly written. Many journals require an abstract structured into objectives, methods, results, and conclusions. Structuring facilitates writing of abstracts and greatly improves their focus.

References and Acknowledgements

Scientific papers should be properly referenced. References must be adequate and follow the style of the journal (e.g. Vancouver, Harvard), and restricted to those with a direct bearing on the work described. It is always advisable to check the journal's instructions and make sure that all necessary details have been included for each reference.

Acknowledgements are contributions to a paper that do not justify authorship. The people acknowledged usually do not take intellectual responsibility for the scientific content of a paper. It is appropriate to acknowledge financial and material support for the research.

Style Matters

Two meanings of the word style are especially relevant to the writing and publishing of scientific articles. Firstly, style means a manner of expression in language. The second meaning is the custom followed by a journal in spelling, capitalization, punctuation, citing references, displays (e.g. figures and tables), and format – the house style.

House style

House style is easier to deal with. Most journals have a distinctive house style that contributes to their identity. Its essentials are given as instructions to authors. Most authors seem to blithely ignore them. They do so at their own peril, because editors tend to favour articles that bear evidence of authors' attention to house style. Editors also prefer short articles without florid prose or redundancies, with short lists of references. Lengthy reference lists do not impress editors, contrary to what some authors seem to think.

General style

Good manner of expression in language is hard to define. The easy way out of this intractable difficulty is to give widely accepted rules of good writing, and examples of clumsy or ungraceful writing. The basic rules of good writing are straightforward: be clear, concise and accurate. Some hints on how these goals can be achieved are given below.

Use the familiar word instead of a far-fetched one, and prefer the short word to a long one. Do not use *accommodation* when *home*, *house* or *flat* would do. *Change* or *alter* may be more appropriate than *diversify*. *Exemplify* is not more impressive than *show*, *illustrate* or *represent*, and *conglomeration* is not more erudite than *collection* or *medley*. *Aetiopathology* and *aetiopathogenesis* should be banned by law. *Cardiac pathological entity* is a silly way of saying *heart disease*.

Prefer the single word to circumlocution. *Did not pay attention to* can be changed to *ignored*, *did not remember* to *forgot*, and *not very important* to *insignificant*. These three examples show also that the positive expression is more assertive than the tame and less effective negative form. Other examples of roundabout expressions, with the single word in parentheses, include: as a result of (because), due to the fact that (since), and at this point in time (now).

Choose the right word. *Disinterested* should not be used to mean *uninterested*. To *refute* a diagnosis is to prove that it is wrong, whereas *repudiate* is to deny, reject or disown utterly, as in "I repudiate that accusation", or "He repudiated the agreement". *Anticipated* and *expected* have different connotations. If a batsman anticipated a googly, he has seen it coming and adjusted his stroke appropriately. If a host has anticipated his guests' needs he must have provided for them in advance.

Beware of a succession of long sentences. Long and complicated sentences increase the chances of confusion about tenses, losing agreement between subjects and verbs, and the syntax going awry. This is not to say that all your sentences ought to be short, only that long ones need careful construction. Varying the length of sentences is, in general, good style. Prefer the active voice, as it has greater impact and immediacy, to the passive construction, which may be quite dull when used often. So "It was observed that ..." is better written as "We observed that ...", and "It became clear that drug A..." is an awfully boring way of saying "Clearly, drug A was better ..."

Avoid jargon and do not use clichés. "The patient *exhibited* the clinical features of ..." Did he actually display them for public viewing? If he didn't, use *had* or *showed* instead of *exhibited*. "The animals were *sacrificed* 24 hours later". Did you do that to invoke the favour of a god? If not, use *killed*. Do not use *expired*, *passed away* or *succumbed* when you mean *died*, *symptomatology* for symptoms, *aetiology* for cause, *wastage* for waste, or *dosage* for dose.

Examples of common clichés include *if and when*, *last but not least* and *in terms of*.

Metaphors are useful to convey ideas succinctly, and often attractively, e.g. ceiling, spearhead, launch, highlight and target. But to use them too frequently or indiscriminately will bring the writer no credit. And mixed metaphors, such as the two well known examples given below, invite hilarity or ridicule depending on the reader's mood.

i.   The sacred cows have come to roost with a vengeance.

ii. I smell a rat, I see it floating in the air; let us nip it in the bud.

If you wish to improve your style, read the chapters dealing with it in the books listed below, learn to subedit your own article, and ask a senior colleague who writes well (the species is rare) to critically assess your style.

References

1.   Hall George M, ed. *How to Write a Paper*. London: BMJ Publishing Group; 1994.

2.   Huth Edward J. *How to Write and Publish Papers in the Medical Sciences*.2nd ed. London: Williams and Wilkins;1990.

3.   Strunk William, White E B. *The Elements of Style*.3rd ed. New York: Macmillan Publishing Co., Inc.; 1979.

4.   Gowers Sir Ernest. (Revised by Greenbaum Sidney, Whitcut Janet). *The Complete Plain Words*. London: Pengin Books; 1986.

5.   Cheryl Iverson (Chair) et al. *American Medical Association Manual of Style*. 9th ed. London, Baltimore, Philadelphia: Williams and Wilkins; 1997.

How to Compile and Write a Thesis

R. Navaratnam

Introduction

Writing a thesis remains one of the biggest non-clinical dilemmas facing surgical trainees or residents during the period of their training. The majority of them, however, embark on this task completely unprepared.

Why Undertake Research?

Why undertake this often laborious and painstaking chore, which often requires numerous drafts, is poorly remunerated and where the scientific impact is often low? There are two primary aims in undertaking research and writing a thesis. In the majority of surgical communities a period of time spent in research (either clinical or laboratory-based) is mandatory to ensure career progress.[1] The other main aim is to increase personal expertise in a sub-specialty area of interest, with a view to critiquing the literature, and thus maintaining a high standard of clinical practice, which is evidence-based. However, it remains a discipline synonymous with the craft of surgery, namely the undertaking of a task which may not always be straightforward, may sometimes go wrong, but largely is immensely rewarding.

Timing of Research

The timing and duration of research within a surgical training programme remains open to discussion and is often left to fate. Ideally, a trainee should commence his higher surgical training programme and then undertake research after 2 years.[1] This enables him to acquire knowledge of some basic surgical techniques and sufficient clinical experience so that he may identify his own particular interests and a potential niche for investigation. The main shortcoming, it may be argued, is that there are disadvantages in leaving regular surgical practice, so early in the surgical apprenticeship. The alternative argument is that it is now often mandatory to possess a higher degree prior to short-listing, in order to enter a higher surgical training programme. Both remain feasible arguments.

What Type of Research Degree?

A minimum of one year of research should be encouraged, with a formal taught component, which should incorporate, as the bare minimum, molecular biology techniques, medical statistics and IT. Computer literacy, ability to use Internet to perform a Medline search and ability to type are the skills which will be increasingly improved during a period of research.

In the UK, the MSc is a one year programme with a significant taught component. This should be sufficient for the majority of British surgical trainees, especially in view of the UK government's drive for modernizing medical careers (MMC) and the proposed consultant expansion programme, with reduced formal training. The two-year MD (or equivalent MS) or the three-year PhD tend to be largely unstructured, but do carry more academic weight in an interview.

Preparation

In order that the research period is a success, careful preparation is essential. Identify a research laboratory, a clinician or a scientist that you are familiar with or want to work with. Prior to meeting him/her, scrutinize his/her research interests. Ask about the form of funding available to support you through your term as a research fellow and enquire (politely) what alternative means would be available, should the initial funding not materialize (which may often be the case).[2]

I routinely recommend that the trainees should ideally have a rough estimation of their projects at least 3-6 months prior to taking up their posts. Due to the widespread introduction of the European working time directive (which may soon be implemented across both sides of the Atlantic), this should be entirely feasible, as the practical surgical teaching decreases, more emphasis may be placed on surgical research. During this period of time they should get familiar with any practical techniques they need to use during their research, in addition to undertaking a literature review. Furthermore, obtaining ethical approval for the work to be undertaken or obtaining an animal licence can also be extremely time consuming.

It is regrettable that a number of trainees start their formal period of research without undertaking any of the above tasks.

Funding

It should be borne in mind that a period of research often represents a significant financial commitment; this is especially true in the absence of a research grant or a regular salary (received in lieu of a regular teaching or clinical commitment).

Obtaining an MRC or Wellcome Trust grant on your own is extremely difficult; however, an application from within an established research unit with a proven academic track record is more likely to be successful.[2]

Experimental Techniques and Laboratory-based Work

It is now evident that the emphasis of surgical research has changed from a patient-orientated approach to a more refined experimental level encompassing new techniques in molecular biology.[3] This has enabled surgical trainees to familiarize themselves with techniques such as the polymerase chain reaction, fundamental to the appreciation of the molecular biology of cancer. This has led to the advancement of modern experimental techniques such as gene therapy, in the modern management of malignancy and other disease processes.[4]

Working with Non-medical Colleagues

Whilst learning either a clinical or a laboratory-based technique, the majority of trainees work in close association with non-clinical or non-medical trained staff, often in a completely alien environment. This relationship needs to be nurtured, because it is almost impossible to progress without their close involvement in the work. In addition, most trainees are so used to an almost regimented day with the routine of outpatients, operating lists, etc. that the often vast expanse of free time is a cause for concern for them. It is advisable to have a regular (weekly) clinical commitment incorporating one outpatient, a day case list and an on-call obligation (preferably at a hospital the trainee is familiar with). This enables some degree of clinical continuity, some financial remuneration and also ensures that the impact of returning to clinical duties, in time, is lessened.

Thesis Layout

The thesis itself should read like a novel, with an introduction and conclusion. One should avoid having a number of experimental chapters which are not well connected with one another. The individual sections should include, an acknowledgements section, an index, an abstract, an introduction, materials and methods (incorporating a section on validation of techniques utilized), a minimum of 3 experimental chapters (preferably 4), a discussion (including a conclusion), an appendix (including all raw data obtained) and a concluding summary of the areas of further potential research. A final page should summarize all published work including that presented at scientific meetings. All references should be accurately documented, as some examiners will check some of them, especially their own.

Acknowledgements, Index and the Abstract

The acknowledgements section is self-explanatory; it should include names of your supervisor and all laboratory and clinical staff that have helped ease the academic burden. The index should represent the overall scheme of the thesis. An abstract, a page in length, should represent an overview of all relevant findings, thus enabling the reader to obtain an overall idea of what is about to unfold.

Writing the Introduction

Writing the introduction is often time consuming. An efficient manner in which this can be undertaken, is by writing a systematic review article which incorporates the majority of your introduction (thus ensuring at least one publication) prior to start of the research period. This often highlights deficiencies in the literature thus directing attention to any potential research opportunities.[5,6]

This aspect of the thesis writing often requires a critical and an efficient appraisal of the literature. A structured format should be undertaken for each individual paper gone through, incorporating a critique of the title, the institution from where the paper originates, inclusion and exclusion criteria used, the validity of the techniques utilized, number of subjects used, the relevance of a power calculation, the appropriateness of the statistics used, the presentation of the data and the validity of the conclusions made in light of the data obtained.

Materials and Methods

Time spent in mastering a new experimental technique is invaluable. Once comfortable with the technique and having validated your data against appropriately validated data (all of which should be published in the appendix section), you can start independent practice of the technique. The advantage of this being data accumulation. In view of the time constraints, this will enable you to accumulate data often 'out of hours', ensuring respectable numbers of subjects in each study.

Experimental Chapters

Traditionally, each experimental chapter has comprised a results section, incorporating numerical and graphical data, followed by discussion and concluding summary sections. However, if each experimental chapter incorporates a new technique, then the more logical approach is to incorporate in each, introduction, independent methodology, results and discussion sections. Enlisting the help of a mature statistician with a good working knowledge of an easily reproducible statistical software package is essential.

The experimental trials may be performed simultaneously. This has significant advantages when performing clinical trials, as on some occasions individual patients may be used in more than one trial, thus minimizing patient inconvenience and also maximizing data accumulation. It must be emphasized how important it is to maintain excellent working relationships with not only your surgical, but also your medical and non-medical colleagues. The former may often give you golden nuggets of information which stimulate areas of further research; alternatively, collaboration with an established unit is an excellent way of nurturing quality data.

The importance of an excellent working relationship with the non-medical staff needs to be re-emphasized as they may often be called upon by you to initiate a particular day's work, especially if you are late following a clinical commitment.

Results and Statistics

Even in the event of not obtaining any credible results, the manner in which the data are presented and have been analyzed remains an extremely important aspect of the assessment of a thesis. The results section should incorporate both the negative and positive findings and these should be tabulated and displayed graphically. It is imperative that the statistical package used is cited, and it is vital that your data are analyzed by an experienced statistician prior to presentation or prior to going to print.

The Discussion

The discussion is inevitably based on the analysis of the results obtained. If written at the end of each chapter, it should be succinct and critical, bearing in mind that an overall discussion will also be written. Aim to have each experimental chapter published independently.

The overall discussion should summarize the relevant positive and significant negative findings. The absence of any "earth shattering" data should not dishearten the trainee; perhaps, of equal relevance is the manner in which the negative data are analyzed.

References and Appendix

Gathering references is often laborious, but the list of references should be built up in a sequential manner. The majority of references will be required during the construction of the introduction and this is the ideal time to amass them, i.e. before you start your actual research.

There are excellent software packages available for accumulating references, such as Reference Manager. A significant advantage of their use is that the references can be automatically formatted according to specifications of the individual journal.[7]

The appendix should incorporate all experimental data obtained (including the initial validation data). This should be in tabulated format and easily referenced to each experimental chapter.

The Role of the Supervisor

The role of a supportive supervisor, who will critique your work in an efficient and sympathetic manner, is important at this stage of writing. It is important at this stage that the turnround of any amendments suggested, is done in an efficient manner in order that these are fresh in your supervisor's mind, as he/she may have more than one thesis to read. A proposed manner in which the thesis should be presented to a supervisor is that following the initial authorization of the introduction and materials and methods sections, individual experimental chapters should be forwarded; however, presentation of the entire thesis (i.e. all the experimental chapters together) may give a supervisor an overall flavour of the message being conveyed.

Presentation

Presenting your data at local, national and international levels is extremely important. On a personal note, the presentation of some preliminary experimental data at a local in-house meeting completely transformed my thesis. Similarly, the personal feedback and criticisms that are obtained from the various scientific fora attended are often invaluable and may shed light on specific areas where there is little information in the literature.

The Thesis Viva

The thesis viva should not represent a huge academic hurdle. Inevitably, a trainee would have spent a minimum of 2-3 years researching a unique field and would thus be well conversant with the literature, the pitfalls associated with the particular thesis and the clinical relevance and the potential implications. The trainee should be conversant with the methodology and the experimental techniques involved as these often remain unfamiliar to the majority of clinicians. A coherent explanation of why certain techniques did not succeed may also be required.

A thesis will never be absolutely perfect; for many, it will represent means to an end. Whilst attempting to be as critical as possible, this must be borne in mind when writing up a thesis. Also, it should be realized that a good quality finished product is more acceptable than 3 unfinished chapters of great excellence.

Conclusion

The emphatic message should be that the entire exercise of writing a thesis is comparable to the art of surgery. There are going to be days when things go very well and there are inevitably days when they don't; and learning to successfully negotiate a large proportion of the perceived problems is synonymous with surgical maturity. The aim should be an overall improvement in the ability to evaluate clinical data, in order to maintain a high standard of clinical practice, which is evidence-based.

References

1. Azmy IAF, Wood D, Reed MWR. Research in surgical training: why, when, where and how? *Ann R Coll Surg Eng (Suppl)*. 2001; 83:341-343.
2. Stebbing J. The advice zone: "How do I get an MD"? *BMJ*. 2004; 15th May.
3. Taylor I. The changing face of surgical research. *Ann R Coll Surg Eng (Suppl)*. 2000; 82:234-235.
4. Williams GL, Ivil KD. Molecular biology research and the trainee surgeon. *Ann R Coll Surg Eng (Suppl)*. 2002; 84:162-163.
5. Sheldon TA. Systematic reviews and meta-analyses: the value for surgery. *Br J Surg*. 1999; 86: 977-978.
6. Egger M, Davey Smith G. Meta-analysis: principles and procedures. *BMJ*. 1998; 315: 1533-7.
7. Cartnell M, Kingsnorth A. Use of the Internet and information technology for surgeons and surgical research. *Ann R Coll Surg Eng*. 2002; 84:352-356.

Critical Appraisal of a Scientific Paper

S. V. Shrikhande & P. J. Shukla

Introduction

There is a lot of research taking place around the world. However, it has been estimated that about one half of research undertaken is misconceived.[1] Quality of a scientific paper is, therefore, the primary responsibility of the authors of the paper. To some extent, a reviewer can contribute to the quality of the paper either during the process of peer review or, after publication, where a scientific paper may draw comments in the correspondence section of a journal.

Scientific significance and originality of a paper are important criteria in judgement of its value. In this chapter we have attempted to provide a broad overview of the process of critical appraisal for the benefit of potential/future reviewers.

Critical Appraisal of a Scientific Paper

Two areas which require attention are originality and scientific content.

Originality of the paper

Most commonly, manuscripts are either clinical or basic science papers. In a clinical paper, the reviewer should investigate whether the author has focused on the efficacy or effectiveness of the particular hypothesis that is being evaluated. Efficacy is the specific outcome under ideal circumstances, whereas effectiveness seeks to determine whether an intervention does more good than harm in patients under normal clinical circumstances. An example is the extent of lymphadenectomy in gastric cancer. To test efficacy one may look only at the success rate of extended lymph node clearance in suitably selected patients. To test effectiveness, however, one will have to consider major outcome measures such as survival and quality of life. Therefore, effectiveness evaluates lymph node clearance, and it may challenge the very concept of extended lymphadenectomy in gastric cancer. Hence, the reviewer must seek to understand why the study was undertaken from the very outset of the process of review.

Scientific Relevance to the Medical and Surgical Community

In the book, *"A Surgeon's Guide to Writing and Publishing"* by Fingerhut et al.,[2] the concept of "taming the literature" has been well described. The reviewer must be critical and ensure that the authors have avoided the temptation of being selective or dismissive of material that contradicts their hypothesis or results. The use of selective bibliography to reinforce a theory should be a strong indication for rejection, or at least a major revision, of a scientific paper.

It is also important to review the historical literature. There is very little original "new" work in medicine today. In this background, it is imperative to view the relevance of the manuscript in its historical context.

After a thorough literature study followed by evaluation of the manuscript, the question the reviewer is expected to ask is "Is all this of any real significance"? To cite a clinical example, a statistical increase in survival with chemotherapy in advanced gall bladder cancer may need to be only a few weeks, but is this really important or worthwhile?

The Finer Details

After the initial broad evaluation of the purpose and relevance of the scientific paper, the reviewer must focus on its finer details. The areas that need consideration are:

1. The Materials and Methods section

How was the study conducted? While prospective, controlled studies are ideal, case studies and part prospective and part retrospective studies are common and they must come lower down in the ladder of scientific merit. The reviewer would be expected to evaluate and understand the particular style of the study and whether the result justifies the hypothesis being tested.

The study population. It is relevant to understand whether a specific population was evaluated or whether the general population was evaluated. In this context, the inclusion and exclusion criteria need to be carefully looked into. A selection bias will invariably result in misleading observations and conclusions. Furthermore, approval from the hospital committee for study of human subjects or animals should be reconfirmed while evaluating this section.

Sample size and methodology. Attention to this important area enables the reviewer to evaluate whether the authors have considered the methods of analysis and necessary sample size before embarking on the study. For example, a small sample size leads to trials with weak power to detect important differences in outcome.

During editorial review of the manuscript this section should be evaluated carefully to determine whether the authors understand the methodology sufficiently to repeat a particular experiment. Often one or more methods described in this section have not been reported previously and will serve as the basis for future laboratory experiments by other investigators. It is important that the reviewer guides the authors to keep this section simple and free of confusion because it often is the foundation for all that follows in the manuscript.

2. The Results and Discussion sections

In the results section, the reviewer must ensure that the results are precise and not repeated in any way. Often, results are written in the form of a description and later tabulated. Also, results should be only those that have some relevance to the study and not necessarily all results that were obtained during the study. Therefore, the reviewer must ensure that the sections describing materials and methods and the discussion are well written, concise and clear, which would automatically ensure crisp presentation of the results.

In the discussion section, the reviewer should evaluate whether an analytical assessment of the results has been provided. It is often noticed that the discussion tends to get wayward with the expression of individual opinions. The reviewer must ensure that a linear link between the material and methods, the results and the discussion sections is maintained. Other areas in the discussion that need attention are whether a comparative analysis with similar studies done in the past has been made. This must be ensured even if data from such studies are conflicting. Authors often do not discuss the shortcomings of their own study and the reviewer should make an effort to highlight these shortcomings and have them incorporated. Such constructive criticism can only improve the overall quality and impact of the scientific paper.

3. Assessment of statistics

Reviewers must be up-to-date with current statistical methods and appropriate use of statistical tests.[3,4] The expert is often able to identify studies in which there has been no prior statistical planning. The reviewer must also ensure that the results of a well designed study are easy to follow and not full of complicated statistics. Generally, powerful results would only require simple statistical tests to make their point. Beware of studies in which complex statistical evaluation has been used. Such a paper may be referred to an expert in statistics, who is usually a member of the review board of a journal.

Critical Appraisal Specific to Some Common Types of Publications

1. Case reports

A case report is often the best way to cut your teeth in scientific writing. Inexperienced authors should be given preference for this type of publication and encouraged to write case reports. The reviewer should make sure that they are brief, adequately illustrated, and convey a truly novel observation, an occurrence that is becoming increasingly uncommon in this era of information explosion.

2. Review articles

The reviewer must ensure that these articles, which review a single topic, provide a broad and adequate overview of the subject. A thorough review of the literature is necessary and the reviewer must evaluate the literature in great detail to ensure that a balanced, practical perspective with current guidelines (in clinical topics) has been provided by the authors to the busy clinician. Currently, meta-analyses are being employed more frequently in provision of scientific guidelines.

3. Original articles

The results of the study should be carefully evaluated. A clear understanding of the data and results will enable the reviewer to evaluate the conclusions drawn. The reviewer must ensure that the conclusions are based solely on the results since authors generally tend to speculate.

4. Technique papers

A reviewer is expected to critically evaluate whether a technique paper really reports some technical aspect that is novel or innovative. The technique should be described with the help of good, clear illustrations and/or photographs. The reviewer must ensure that adequate clinical experience is documented to justify the technique described. Unless the technique is truly novel, description of such a technique in isolated patients should be discouraged.

5. Basic research articles

In the times when basic science papers are dominating an increasing number of journals, even some editors believe that basic research papers have more inherent value and worth than clinical papers. A journal with a balanced proportion of basic science and clinical papers would be attractive to all in the scientific community. Ultimately, basic science must be a means to an end. Hence, an important goal of reviewers of basic science work is to ensure that the science being reported will have clinical relevance. But, good science remains good science and bad science is bad science irrespective of where it is published.[2, 5]

Summary

It is the responsibility of the reviewers to guide and help the authors to improve their scientific work. To this end they must evaluate the scientific article purely on the basis of its educational content and its relevance to current medical science. They must not allow other factors (conflict of interest, seniority of the author, etc.) to affect the process of decision making. Reviewers must remember they have a great responsibility towards the readers as well as the authors, who have entrusted their scientific work to the journal.

In the critical appraisal of a scientific paper, reviewers must recognize what authors expect from editors and reviewers: they solicit serious analysis of the submissions, fairness and balance, absence of conflict of interest, openness to new ideas and willingness to perform timely reviews. It is worth remembering that every reviewer will in turn be an author, in need of good review.[6]

References

1. Horton R. Surgical research or comic opera: Questions but few answers. *Lancet*. 1996;347:984.

2. Schein M, Farndon JR, Fingerhut A, eds. *A Surgeon's Guide to Writing and Publishing*. United Kingdom: Blackwell Science; 2001.

3. Murray GD. Statistical aspects of research methodology. *Br J Surg*.1991;78:777-81.

4. Murray GD. Statistical guidelines for the British Journal of Surgery. *Br J Surg*. 1991;78:782-84.

5. Sarr MG. Generating an idea: will it be publishable? *Br J Surg*. 2000;87:388-89.

6. Warshaw AL. What an editor wants or expects from authors (commentary). In: Schein M, Farndon JR, Fingerhut A, eds. *A Surgeon's Guide to Writing and Publishing*. United Kingdom: Blackwell Science; 2001: 131-132.

Research Misconduct

Stewart A. Laidlaw

The conduct of science is based on trust. One of the major reasons for public trust in, and funding of, science is the belief that the way science is conducted is honest and ethical. Loss of that public trust would be a catastrophe for the progress of scientific research. Therefore, it is crucial that, as a scientist, you hold yourself to the highest standards of ethical conduct. We are all human beings, however, and subject to the pressures and temptations that afflict everyone. We are also human in the way that we seek patterns and hold to prejudices that are non-scientific, to the detriment of science. It is important for us to be aware of our failings and to guard against them at all times.

Most of the articles written about research misconduct tend to focus on the more spectacular examples of "scientists gone bad" and there is ample literature on, and case studies about, individual scientists who have, for various reasons, found it necessary to engage in research misconduct. This chapter will focus only briefly on these matters since, although instructive, they may be aberrant and not representative of the kinds of unethical conduct that may be more pervasive and less acknowledged in the practice of science.

In that context, there are a number of high profile cases that demonstrate examples of these major definitions and the consequences for individuals, and for society as a whole, of research misconduct.

The Summerlin case,[1] involving falsification of skin graft results by marking white mice with black marker illustrates the tragic personal consequences of pressure to produce positive results. The case of

John Darsee[2,3,4] points out the potential for affecting the lives and careers of colleagues by involving them in publications in which data were fabricated; it also points out the responsibility of co-authors to check and then stand by data to which they lend their names. The circumstances surrounding Dr. Robert Slutsky, then at UC San Diego, demonstrate that wholesale fabrication of data can be used to further an academic career; Dr. Slutsky's phenomenal publication output (one paper every ten days over the course of several years) ultimately put a major research university on its mettle, to which it responded in an exemplary manner.[5]

In the wider context of the effects of research misconduct on society, Stephen Breuning's publication of fabricated data on psychoactive drugs (including Ritalin) for the treatment of psychiatric disorders[6,7] had a profound effect on prescribing practices and public health policies nationwide and led to considerable distrust of such research, while probably exposing thousands of subjects to risk on the basis of experiments not performed.

Finally, the case of Werner Bezwoda from South Africa[8,9,10] illustrates the considerable financial and economic consequences of research misconduct, to say nothing of the toll in human suffering and false hope that resulted from the dissemination of false research results on treatment of breast cancer. In addition, a potentially promising field of research has probably been tainted forever by the fallout from this betrayal of the public trust.

These examples illustrate why research misconduct is so damaging; not only does it affect individuals and their colleagues, but society as a whole can suffer from the negative consequences of reliance on tainted research. In turn, public trust in science is diminished and the scientific enterprise suffers. The more prominent cases, and the publicity they have attracted, however, have led to the development of standards of conduct that we all live under, so it is instructive to consider them.

Currently, the U.S. government has defined certain areas of conduct that are considered unacceptable in the practice of science. The current definition of research misconduct[11] is:

Research misconduct is defined as fabrication, falsification, or plagiarism in proposing, performing, or reviewing research, or in reporting research results.

- *Fabrication* is making up data or results and recording or reporting them.
- *Falsification* is manipulating research materials, equipment, or processes, or changing or omitting data or results such that the research is not accurately represented in the research record.
- *Plagiarism* is the appropriation of another person's ideas, processes, results, or words without giving appropriate credit.
- Research misconduct *does not include* honest error or differences of opinion.

Fabrication, falsification and plagiarism are three different aspects of the same desire to seek positive results. They differ only in the degree of difficulty. In the case of falsification, it is necessary to actually conduct the experiment and then to "fix" the data to correspond to your preconceived notions of what is correct. In the second, fabrication, you avoid all the time, effort and messiness of actually conducting the experiments, by just creating a dataset to correspond to your preconceived notions of what is correct. Plagiarism is the easiest of all; avoid all the intellectual effort to make up numbers by just appropriating the ideas of others and passing them off as your own. This may seem a flippant way to address the issue, but it illustrates the point.

Plagiarism is probably the research misconduct you would be most likely to fall prey to, and usually inadvertently. Cases of wholesale appropriation of others' ideas, data, written words, etc. are not common[12,13] but often are relatively easy to detect because the appropriated material often looks "different" from the material surrounding it, or because many people are reading the literature and comparing the ideas presented. In the field of academic research, however, you are likely to read and think about all of the major work in the field you choose to work in, so inevitably you will be exposed to the ideas and words of your colleagues over an extended period of time. When you come to write up your own work for publication, you will refer to the previous work by others, with appropriate attribution (see the References section at the end of this article, for example); what happens, however, when a particularly felicitous turn of phrase from another researcher's paper sticks in your mind? How easy is it to forget when writing your own article where that sentence that aptly describes a phenomenon comes from? Probably very easy, and, therefore, it is all the more reason to consider carefully everything that you write. It should go without saying that data and ideas communicated to you in confidence (for example, as a reviewer for a journal, or as a member of a study section) should be treated as confidential and not exploited without attribution of the source.

When you embark upon a research career, you are likely to confidently assert that you would never resort to large scale fabrication, falsification or plagiarism, and you are probably correct; nevertheless, in many smaller ways you may find yourself tempted to behaviour that is outside acceptable norms in science. It is important to be aware of how easily this can happen and to guard against it.

One of the main problems you may encounter is not thinking closely about what you are actually trying to do when you conduct an experiment, test a device or technique or evaluate an investigational drug in a clinical trial. All of these are exercises meant to test a hypothesis (Drug A is better than Drug B; this newer surgical technique results in fewer complications than the current accepted technique, etc.). Most people talk about conducting experiments to prove a hypothesis and in casual language "prove" has come to mean "showing that it is true". In fact, however, the scientific use of "prove" means to "test" a hypothesis, in other words, to put your hypothesis to the test to see whether it measures up. Experiments are designed to see if your hypothesis correctly predicts the results. Consequently, the data that are often most useful to you as a practicing scientist are the data that do not "fit" with your hypothesis, because these are the data that are challenging your hypothesis. The temptation is to disregard these data if they do not conform to your pre-existing notion of how things should "be". This is easy to do – you assume that something went wrong and that the data in question are wrong. It is a human trait to wish to see positive outcomes; it is equally human to want to hold on to a cherished idea that you expended a lot of effort and thought to come up with. In fact, however, if the experiment was conducted appropriately and if you recorded your data comprehensively, and none of the conditions was aberrant, then you are obliged to accept the results, however contradictory they may be to your expected outcome. This is sometimes tough to do, but it is necessary to always be willing to discard or modify your hypothesis in the face of evidence to the contrary. In fact, the contrary result should be a cause for celebration, because it reminds you that all hypotheses are provisional and subject to change.

Another problem you may encounter is the all too human wish to see patterns in data, even where patterns may not exist. Consider the following two sets of data (Figs 14.1 and 14.2):

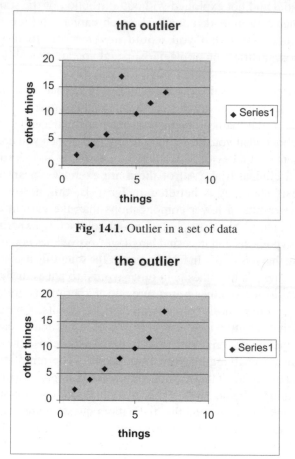

Fig. 14.1. Outlier in a set of data

Fig. 14.2. Outlier in a set of data

In the first figure, there appears to be a linear relationship between the values on the X-axis and those on the Y-axis, with the exception of one "outlier". Inclusion of this datum in the correlation will lead to a straight line correlation that does not pass through any of the points on the graph; the temptation would be to ignore the "outlier" to attain a better fit of the data. Notice, however, in the second plot, the same data points are plotted; the only difference is the placement of the "outlier". In this case, I suggest that most people would be satisfied with the general run of the data points and would accept the "outlier"; context is often everything, but if one would not accept the "outlier" in the first graph, why would it be more acceptable in the second?

It is also important to remember that in any experiment, you are looking to test the null hypothesis – the hypothesis that there **is no** difference between the two sets of conditions you are comparing or between the two sets of data you have generated. Using statistical methods, you assess the likelihood that the differences you **do** observe might have arisen by random chance; it is only when the statistical probability that these differences are due to random variation is very low that you allow yourself to be dragged, kicking and screaming, to the conclusion that the differences are real. So, in any experiment, the approach should be one of skepticism about the data; only as a last resort should you be willing to accept that the differences are real. Unfortunately, many novice researchers approach the problem from exactly the opposite direction.

Another critical judgment to be made, even after demonstrating to your satisfaction that you have a "real" difference, is in judging whether that difference is of any clinical utility; many experiments can show statistical differences between two different drug regimens or the outcome of two different surgical procedures. In the real world, however, does this difference lead to a significant improvement in patient care? This, after all, is why academic physicians are in the business of doing research in the first place – to improve patient care.

Finally, science progresses by small steps, building on the work of those who have gone before; therefore, it is more realistic to seek small, but significant, improvements in treatment, rather than grand re-workings of current practice. Current practice did not become current practice without some basis in fact (one would hope). Having said that, however, you should always be on the lookout for practices implemented on the basis of preconceived notions, cultural prejudice, etc.; this is more common in science than is generally admitted.

What is your responsibility if you come across something that appears to be research misconduct, as defined above? Your responsibility as a scientist is to ensure that data are reported accurately. If there is a question, you must raise it; loyalty to colleagues, fear of being considered a "snitch", consideration of deference to a more senior colleague must all be put aside. The strength of science is in its integrity. If something undermines that integrity, it casts doubt on all of science. Most institutions have mechanisms in place to handle questions in a systematic way, via an Ethics Committee or some other mechanism and there are protections for whistleblowers to try to ensure that all research misconduct investigations are handled with minimum consequences to those who raise issues.

References

1. Culliton BJ. The Sloan-Kettering affair: a story without a hero. *Science.*1974; 184: 644-650.
2. Broad WJ. Harvard delays in reporting fraud. *Science.* 1982; 215: 478-482.
3. Broad WJ. Report absolves Harvard in case of fakery. *Science* 215 (1982) 874-876
4. Culliton BJ. The Darsee case. *Science.* 1983; 220: 31-35.
5. Marshall E. San Diego's tough stand on research fraud. *Science.* 1986; 234: 534-535.
6. Holden C. NIMH review of fraud charges moves slowly. *Science.* 1986; 234: 1488-1489.
7. Holden C. Breuning's accuser has grant deferred. *Science.* 1987; 236: 145.
8. Hagmann M. Cancer researcher sacked for alleged fraud. *Science.* 2000; 287: 1901-1902.
9. Weiss RB, Rifkin RM, Stewart FM, Theriault RL, Williams LA, Herman AA, Beveridge RA. High-dose chemotherapy for high-risk primary breast cancer: an on-site review of the Bezwoda study. *Lancet.* 2000; 355: 999-1003.
10. Horton R. After Bezwoda. *Lancet.* 2000; 355: 942-943.
11. Code of Federal Regulations 42 CFR 93.103 (2005).
12. Broad WJ. Would be academician pirates papers. *Science.* 1980; 208 (1): 1438-1440.
13. Broad WJ. Charges of piracy follow Alsabti. *Science.* 1980; 210: 291.

Index